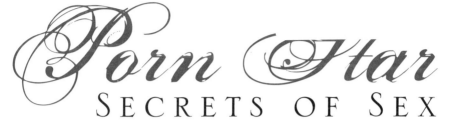

SECRETS OF SEX

OVER **100** MIND-BLOWING
TIPS, TRICKS, AND GAMES
YOU WISH YOU KNEW

JENI WEST

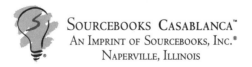

SOURCEBOOKS CASABLANCA™
AN IMPRINT OF SOURCEBOOKS, INC.®
NAPERVILLE, ILLINOIS

Copyright © 2008 by Sourcebooks, Inc.
Cover and internal design © 2008 by Sourcebooks, Inc.
Sourcebooks and the colophon are registered trademarks of Sourcebooks, Inc.

All rights reserved. No part of this book may be reproduced in any form or by any electronic or mechanical means including information storage and retrieval systems—except in the case of brief quotations embodied in critical articles or reviews—without permission in writing from its publisher, Sourcebooks, Inc.

Published by Sourcebooks Casablanca, an imprint of Sourcebooks, Inc.
P.O. Box 4410, Naperville, Illinois 60567-4410
(630) 961-3900
Fax: (630) 961-2168
www.sourcebooks.com

Printed and bound in Canada
TR 10 9 8 7 6 5 4 3 2 1

Contents

Introduction: Naked Ambition v
How to Use Porn Star Ambition to Enhance Your Sex Life

Chapter One: Beauty and the Beast 1
How to Be Beautiful While You Let Out Your Inner Tiger

Chapter Two: Sensual Seduction 15
How to Seduce Your Lover with Foreplay Frenzy

Chapter Three: Going Down to Pleasure Town 39
How to Follow the Map to the Most Delicious Oral Sex
Your Mouth Has Ever Tasted

Chapter Four: The Vintage Collection 53
How to Use Classic Porn Moves to Spice Up Your Sex
Life in the 21st Century

Chapter Five: Forbidden Fruits..............................71
How to Indulge in the Tantalizing Taboo of Fetishes

Chapter Six: Cumming Home 87
How to Get a Happy Ending

Chapter Seven: Titillating and Tantalizing Toys..........103
How to Share Your Sex Toys and Play Well with Others

Chapter Eight: Director's Cut..................................119
How to Sort out the Good, the Bad, and the Very, Very Sexy

Chapter Nine: The Ultimate Visual Stimulation..........127
How to Enjoy a Feast for Four Eyes

Naked Ambition

For generations we have looked up to women like Margaret Mead, Elizabeth Cady Stanton, and Susan B. Anthony as role models to inspire us to ride the equal rights movement by the horns and never look back. We've proudly marched for the ability to vote, burned our bras, and petitioned for our rights, all in defiance of society standards. But is it at the expense of our sexuality?

Many American women still are ashamed of their bodies, begging their lovers to turn off the lights before their trysts, and staying tightly entwined like cocoons in the bed sheets afterward. Why is it that we are more ashamed of our bodies as we grow more confident in our intelligence? And more importantly, who will be the role models to inspire us to embrace our inner sexual self? Who will give us the confidence to take the sexual high road, strip for our lovers, and shine naked in the limelight?

Porn stars.

Adult film actresses are unabashedly unashamed of their bodies, showcasing them to millions of viewers and relishing every minute of it. They embrace their sexuality instead of shunning it. And they exude a carnal confidence that no man can resist. What are their secrets to not only keeping their cool, but also increasing their confidence, as each layer of clothing falls to the floor? How do they bring their lovers to new levels of excitement each day and night without falling into a mediocre lights-out, missionary position rut?

Porn stars know the tips, rules, and how-to's on sex because sex is their job, their career, and their livelihood. More importantly, they have the trade secrets of great, mind-blowing sex because this job is evaluated by millions of viewers daily. That kind of performance anxiety may crack corporate America, but these performing artists relish the attention and have become sex experts because of it.

It's time we took a lesson from these silver screen vixens and became confident, sensual showstoppers on our own.

Beauty and the Beast

 HOW TO BE BEAUTIFUL WHILE YOU
LET OUT YOUR INNER TIGER

Getting sexy isn't about becoming a different person. It's about discovering and displaying what already lies inside of you.

—Brynne Dearie (infamous L.A. stripper)

In our society, women yearn to learn movie stars' tips and secrets on how to get that beautiful, glowing skin, those deep sultry eyes, and that killer body. But notice that when it comes time for most tinsel-town sex scenes, the camera always shies away. We either get a sneak peek at a body part (usually a body double), or a shot of the next morning, with the actors looking gorgeous lying under thousand-thread-count Egyptian cotton sheets.

Porn stars know real beauty secrets because they know how to stay sultry and sexy as they are being filmed getting down and dirty. Who better to learn the tricks of the trade from than the stars who have mesmerized our boyfriends, our husbands, and us, so long into the night? These previously untapped beauty sources have plenty of ideas to offer. Let's explore some head-to-toe tips and secrets for staying sexy while in the sack.

SEXY HEAD-TO-TOE

Smoking Hot Eyes

This look is not for just porn divas, strippers, and A-list celebrities. It's for the sex goddess inside each of us.

- Line the inner rim of your eye with a black or brown eye pencil. Blend only the far edges into your lash line with a cotton swab.
- With a small angled brush, edge a frosty white or pink powder shadow into the inner corner of your eyelid. This will brighten your eyes and also add a dramatic contrast to the black liner.
- With another small angled brush, edge a dark-colored shadow on your bottom lashes and the top of your eyelid.
- Apply mascara to only the tips of your lashes. Then, with a second application, apply to the entire length of your lashes. This will add dramatic volume to your lashes.

You'll drive your lover into such a frenzy with these bedroom eyes that he won't be able to wait until you reach the bed to take you. The smoky hot eye look is dark and shadowed, as if you just had a wild sex romp, smudged your makeup, and are so hungry for more that you don't have time for a touch-up. For added dramatic effect, add some long false eyelashes.

How to Apply Sex Appeal with Faux Eyelashes

Faux eyelashes are making a sexy comeback! Now you can purchase faux lashes that let you apply individual lashes instead of an entire row, for a unique glam look. They even sell faux lashes with tiny gemstones on the ends, for a sparkling experience.

Shush!—here's a little secret on how to apply them without making a mess of your makeup. Apply the adhesive to the lashes, then wait thirty seconds before you apply them to your lash line. This allows the glue to get tacky first, and eliminates the chance of any glue dripping onto your face during application.

Give Him Lip Service

Lips are hailed as one of the most sensual and provocative parts of a woman. They can give large amounts of pleasure and can speak the naughtiest of words. However, with the correct amount of porn-star intuition, you can get your lover all worked up without opening your lips at all.

Heighten his anticipation and excitement with a tinted gloss on your lips. It not only brings attention to the fullness of your mouth and all the delicious things it can do, but the shiny gloss also conjures images of his cum and how beautiful it would look on your lips. All these tantalizing thoughts running through his naughty mind are enough to make him hard even before your mouth starts getting down and dirty.

For added effect, try a new little item that packs a huge punch. A new product called Lip Venom gloss uses spicy ingredients like cinnamon and ginger to increase the circulation in your lips to achieve a flushed, plumped look. It's a great way to get dramatic results quickly without the pain of surgery or injections. Fuller lips also give the appearance of youth and fertility, something all men are innately drawn to.

Nail-Me Nails

The porn industry has transformed the French manicure, elevating it from a fashion couture icon to something a little racier. The image of those perfect white-striped fingernails stroking a hard penis or rubbing a clean pussy is enough to get anyone's juices running. The style has become associated with porn stars, and the sight of them alone can make your lover beg for your touch.

And don't forget your feet! Make sure you get a pedicure, too, so your feet look great when you're getting some mutual satisfaction in the 69 position.

Every porn-star beauty needs a little pampering session. So to get these luscious looks, always make sure you take time out of your busy schedule to treat yourself to some spa treatments. Having a professional do your manicure and pedicure will not only provide some much-needed relaxation time, it will also assure that your nails look great. And while you're there, you can squeeze in an eyebrow wax or back massage; whatever suits your fantastic fancy.

And as an added bonus, your lover will know that if you take such good care of your own appendages, you're likely to shower his with the same attention to delicious detail.

While we've previously been looking at classic beauty tips vamped up with a sexy twist, the next sets of tips are hard-core scarlet secrets about how to let your naughty bits glow in the consummation limelight.

That Banging Body

Many porn stars suggest using cosmetics on some of your most delicious body parts. However, if you are adding definition to those parts, you generally are asking for them to be licked, sucked, and fucked. So for the consideration of your lover, keep all that bronzer at a minimum.

Brazen Breasts

Your breasts are a sizzling source of pleasure for both you and your lover. So put those dirty pillows on a pedestal where they belong by indulging in a little precoital pampering.

Exfoliate: Use the same exfoliator that you use for the rest of your body on your breasts. This will slough off any perspiration, dead skin cells, and tiny bumps on your boobs and leave the skin there smooth and supple. Remember, only exfoliate twice a week. Too many sessions may irritate your skin.

Moisturize: Apply moisturizing lotion to your breasts to hydrate your skin.

Tweeze: Remove any unwanted hairs around your areolae by tweezing them away. Never shave or wax hair in that area. Shaving will cause ingrown hairs. Besides, having a blade in such proximity to your nipples is way too close for anyone's comfort, and waxing is too painful for the delicate skin on your breasts.

Enhance: Dust nipples lightly with a bronzer. This will draw your lover's attention to the focal point of your breasts. Also, many sex-toy parties and online services now offer a gloss you can apply to your nipples that tastes like raspberry, strawberry, or other flavors to titillate your lover's racy taste buds. The gloss also has a secret ingredient that tickles the many nerve endings in your nipples. It's win-win stimulation for everyone involved!

> While the porn industry often opts for the surgical route to obtaining larger breasts, here's a secret for enhancing your oomph naturally without the nip or the tuck. To better define a smaller bust, lightly dust your cleavage with a radiant shimmer powder. The light will reflect off the powder and give an illusion of depth.

How to Get a Smooth Stomach

The stomach is a trouble area for many women. In fact, many hide in the missionary position because they think that if they are on their back, it will flatten their stomach. Rise above that myth, follow the tips below, and climb on top of your lover in triumph!

- First and foremost, before sex, avoid eating or drinking anything that causes you to bloat, such as carbonated drinks, raw veggies, or beans.
- After making coffee in the morning, mix coffee grounds with lotion or oil and rub onto your stomach in a circular motion. Wait several minutes and then rinse clean. The grounds act as an exfoliator, and the caffeine helps get fat cells moving to get rid of cellulite. Do this twice a week for the best results.
- Try belly dancing. Classes are becoming more popular, or you can always pick up a book or DVD and practice in the privacy of your own home. This dance technique will help

tone your stomach muscles and also help you develop a seductive striptease to perform for your lover.

Get Me Some Booty

For those of us who look deep within ourselves and find animalistic tendencies to get down-and-dirty doggy style, the appearance of our derrieres is of the utmost importance. Here are some helpful tips for keeping your bottom in tip-top shape.

- Place your back flush against a wall, with your feet positioned hip-distance apart. Hold your hands straight out in front of you. Slowly slide down the wall until you are in a sitting position. Hold this position for ten seconds, then slowly rise. Repeat this five times. This exercise will dramatically change your butt's shape in just a few weeks' time.
- Drink plenty of water. By quenching your thirst with water, you are actively attacking the unwanted fat that clings to your butt. Plus, water energizes your skin and your body—and with the ass you'll end up with, you'll need that energy to quench your lover's lust.
- Massaging your butt and thighs is a heavenly way to reduce the appearance of cellulite. However, you must do it on a regular basis for the results to last. While most of us may not have the cash for the indulgence of a masseuse, there are a few ways to treat ourselves. Invest in a handheld massager, do a self-massage, or have your lover massage you as part of some delicious foreplay.

The Legs He'll Long For

The flawless appearance of gams in porn films, digitally enhanced with the help of air-brushing porn editors, is hard to achieve at home. But don't worry, porn stars have some secrets up their sleeves on how to get legs so smooth that you can wrap them around your lover's neck, back, and anywhere else you desire, with no inhibitions.

- Always exfoliate legs before shaving. This will remove dead skin cells and bumps, so your skin will be smooth before the razor hits it and will stay smooth afterward.
- Shave with a quality men's razor. They are typically better than ones sold specifically for women because they have multi blades for a smoother shave. Never use a disposable razor.
- Once out of the shower but before you shave, apply an antiperspirant to your legs, either spray or semisolid. This will prevent razor bumps. And always moisturize right after shaving. This will hold in the moisture from your shower and keep your legs soft and supple.

The Nether Regions

Bedhead hair is sexy. Bedhead pubic hair is not. Porn stars know how delicious a Brazilian wax looks and feels, and how well it seduces. However, if you're not brazen enough to try this new trend, there are other fun ways to make the same sensual statement without going totally bare. Think about doing a partial trimming, and take these shapes into consideration.

- **The Heart:** Show your man the depth of your love!
- **The Landing Strip:** Or just show him the way!
- **The Arrow:** A less subtle way to give him a little direction!

· **The Star:** To emphasize the sex star you are!

· **The X:** To showcase how racy you'd like to get!

For an added level of intimacy and trust, have your lover shave you by following these simple steps.

1. Pubic hair is naturally coarse. Soften your hair by taking a sensual bath with your lover before shaving.

2. You or your lover can draw the desired shape with a lip or eyeliner pencil. You can also find stencil kits specifically geared for this racy endeavor online or in adult bookstores. However, if either of you have artistic tendencies, you can draw freehand!

3. Apply shaving cream or conditioner to the area you plan to shave. Both will soften the hair and make it easier to shave.

4. Pull the skin taut, not only to make it easier to shave, but to also ensure the desired shape will have smooth edges.

5. Always use a new blade in this nether region, and shave in the direction that the hair grows. Going against the grain can cause irritation and bumps.

6. Rinse the area. Some shaving creams can leave behind residue that if not thoroughly rinsed, may cause bumps and clogged pores. Not sexy!

CARNAL CONFIDENCE

Now that you have some secrets for staying sexy between the sheets, it's time to find the porn-star confidence to emerge from those sheets and strut your stuff.

How to Seductively Take It All Off

Ask your lover what their number one fantasy is, and you more than likely will get a racy reply involving a tantalizing striptease. The act of seductively taking off one's clothes has for centuries been a visual that men and women alike can't get enough of.

However, those with more experience know all about the *art* of the striptease. One doesn't simply jump out of one's clothes. One must gyrate, swivel, and thrust them to the ground, to highlight the pure thrill of nakedness.

There is a technique to baring it all in the name of art, sex, and love. Follow these steps, bring your lover's favorite fantasy to life, and indulge your inner exhibitionist.

- Always take each item of clothing off tantalizingly slowly. This is why it is called a strip*tease*. Use music to have something to move to (or just use the rhythm of your lover's heavy breathing).
- Take off sweaters and shirts first. Simply roll them over your head and toss them to the side. If you have a button-down shirt, even better! Undo each button slowly, then slip the shirt below your shoulders, and turn your back and let it fall to the ground. (Remember to unbutton the cuffs beforehand so they don't get stuck.)
- With your back to your lover, push your pants or skirt down slowly over your bottom. Be sure to stick your butt out as you do this, and turn your head to see his reaction. After the clothing is beyond your butt, shimmy until it hits the floor. Then just seductively step out of it.
- Turn to face your lover again. Start playing with the straps of

your bra as if you are taking it off. Do this for as long as your lover can take it before you unclasp your bra. However, hold your bra in place. Turn around, and then let your bra fall to the ground. Then turn back to your lover.

- In the same way you teased your lover with taking off your bra, begin playing with your panties. Move them lower and lower. Then stop. Do this as long as you desire. Then turn around, move them over your butt for your lover to view, and shimmy out of them until they hit the floor. As a bonus, let your panties fall to one foot and then kick them off.

- If you have problems removing any item of clothing, have your lover lend a helping hand.

> Wear a thong under panties for some additional teasing!

Flaunt that Confidence

Porn stars ooze sex appeal because they exude a carnal confidence, not only about their bodies but also about their techniques and their very selves. They transcend insecurities to find bliss and happiness in being naked in front of millions of viewers.

You only need to find a fraction of that confidence to be comfortable naked in front of your lover. So what's their secret formula for confidence? To find the porn-star sex goddess within you, simply subtract body hang-ups, add in that humans are naturally more beautiful naked (clothes distort our natural shapes), and multiply by a belief in yourself.

Here are some other ways to add to your own carnal confidence ...

- When you get out of the shower in the morning, stand in front of the mirror and repeat, "I'm beautiful, I'm sexy, I deserve fabulous sex." This mantra will program your mind to believe what is already the truth.
- On days your confidence hits a low, wear something that makes you feel sexy. Get a faux tan, wear some scorching lingerie, or strap on your stilettos. Then request that your lover take a longer-than-usual time revving up your engine with foreplay. The knowledge that he loves touching you will boost your ego.
- Always remember: Having the confidence to try something new in bed is sexy in itself.

It's All in the Lighting

If you're somewhat shy about saddling up with all lights ablaze, but still want to have a randy romp porn-star style, you have a few options.

- **Candlelight:** It is a known fact that all women look beautiful by candlelight, so turn off the lights and use flames to fire up your sex life. You will enjoy the fact that the shadows the candles create will soften the look of your skin, and your man will love actually seeing your curves.
- **Pink Lighting:** Pink tinted light bulbs are the most becoming to all skin tones and cast the most attractive shadows. They hide cellulite, stretch marks, and any other imperfections you may think you have. Other colors that have a similar effect: orange, purple, or red.

Lights Not to Use

- **Pure White Light:** This light is too harsh. It can highlight any flaws you are trying to cover up, and it isn't much of a mood setter.
- **Fluorescent:** This type of light also has a harsh tint and can make you look otherworldly. ET is *not* sexy, no matter how many Oscars he won.

Barely Baring It

Porn stars even have a solution for those who are a little too shy to bare it all. Keep one of the following items on during your racy romp whenever you're not comfortable taking it *all* off. Not only will you have a heightened sense of confidence, but also the vixen visual will thrill your lover.

- **Stilettos:** A sexy woman's favorite accessory; a classic touch to spice things up.
- **Garter Belt and Stockings:** The idea alone is enough to make him stand at attention.
- **Tattoos:** Play up your wild side by giving a twist against your conservative nature.
- **Wigs:** Reach a higher level of role-playing. You're still you, but your hair belongs to the wild woman from the strip club. Go curly, go pink, go crazy.
- **Pasties:** A nice surprise at the end of a naughty striptease (even more so if they have tassels).
- **Lace-up Corset:** Play up your womanly curves.

See It to Believe It!

Want to see how sexy a striptease can be, without leaving the comfort of your home? Watch this fantastic porn film featuring Nina Hartley for some visual pointers.

The Bridal Shower—directed by Candida Royalle, 1997, 80 minutes

Bonus Tip: Always remember: Don't bother obsessing about perceived body flaws. When you lose yourself in each other's pleasure, you'll see just how beautiful being naked really is.

Sensual Seduction

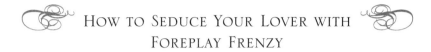 How to Seduce Your Lover with
Foreplay Frenzy

> Seduction is always more singular and
> sublime than sex.
>
> —Jean Baudrillard

While porn may be all about the sizzling sex on screen, when a
porn vixen gets busy between her own sheets, foreplay comes
way before fornication on her scandalous scale of importance.

Don't get those silver-screen divas wrong—they're all about
doing the horizontal tango as often as they can. But they also
know that foreplay is the be-all and end-all of great sex and that
without this erotic element, sex would just be intercourse without
the pop, sizzle, and fireworks.

In a recent study in *The Journal of Sex Research*, it was discovered
that foreplay generally lasts only 11 to 13 minutes. Porn stars
united are shouting at the top of their lungs—they need it
longer, harder, and more creative!

As great foreplay sexperts, porn stars know how to get
what they want. They understand that you must fully
indulge in the sensual before you can fully enjoy the sexual.
Their sensual foreplay collection fully stimulates each one

of the human senses, and it can help you get what you want from sex.

With all their tips, tricks, and titillating tidbits up your sleeve, you'll be able to raise the unacceptable foreplay average while raising your lover's cock at the same time! It makes perfect sex sense!

FOR YOUR VIEWING PLEASURE

Silver-screen vixens understand that seduction and foreplay are not limited to kissing and touching alone but can include a colorful variety of delights that will provide complete satisfaction if done correctly. So follow their lead and set your own sex life ablaze with these sensual foreplay basics.

It's a well-known fact that men are very visual creatures (which may explain why the porn industry is always booming), but it is time to lay to rest the rumor that women are not. Sight can inspire lust in any female's mind and body—a glimpse of her lover's cock peeking in and out between her legs, the sight of her favorite baseball player's ass in those tight pants, even a foxy porn star dressed in her best getup can get a woman's engine revving.

Both genders can rise to the carnal occasion with some presex sightseeing. Try out some of these trade secrets and see how you can use this subtle but very powerful stimulation to your own foreplaying advantage.

Eye Candy

Sometimes even the simplest cliché can seduce your lover into a frenzy. Put on one of the following outfits for your lover after you both have had a long, stressful day at work. Not only will it be a source of visual stimulation for him, but you'll also feel confident and sexy knowing you're a sight for his sore eyes.

- Naughty Nurse
- Innocent School Girl
- French Maid
- Provocative Teacher
- Seducing Secretary
- Angel
- Porn Star
- Police Officer

Some articles of clothing just scream sex and can give him the arousing image he's itching for. Wear one or more of these in the morning (making sure your lover is aware you're sporting these sexy accessories just for him) and he'll have sex on his mind all day!

- Garter Belts
- Teddies
- Pasties
- Stilettos
- Knee-High Boots
- Mini Skirts

For those of you with mega sex goddess style, try combining a miniskirt, a very tight-fitting shirt, and knee-high boots for the ultimate Come-Fuck-Me look.

> Even jewelry can be a sizzling sight! Wear a belly ring or pendant that grazes your cleavage to call attention to these areas. You'll be sure to see a sparkle in his eye.

Look but Don't Touch

Another way to seduce each other with sight is by playing a little game of "you can look, but you cannot touch." Allowing your lover to ravish you with his eyes will give you the boost of confidence to strut your sexy stuff and the knowledge that he can't touch you will rev up his lust. Plus, you can even incorporate some fun light bondage to make it kinky.

Here are a few naughty suggestions on how get the fire started.

- **Clean House:** Walk around the house in your sexiest under-things and stilettos, bend over and pick things up in front of him, sit seductively across from him. Caress your breasts, your thighs, and every delicious place in between. Make sure he sits on his hands for this one.
- **Drop It Like It's Hot:** Dance seductively in front of him in your shortest skirt and tallest boots. If you feel inclined, start to strip each layer off to the beat. You may want to handcuff him to the bed to keep his hands from wandering.
- **A Nice Hot Meal:** Cook an exotic meal wearing only your apron. Set the table and open the wine. Remind him he can watch and learn but can't get any hands-on experience.
- **Wake-Up Call:** Flash your lover a glimpse of your bra and panties before you both head off to work. His testosterone is at a peak in these early morning hours, and the visual will stay with him all day long.

> Another visual treat: Greet him at the door after work clad in nada!

Forbidden Sights

What feels more forbidden and illicit then watching your lover doing simple daily activities without his knowledge? Sneak a peek at your partner showering, getting dressed and undressed, even masturbating in private. The knowledge that you are spying on such innocent scenes will conjure up some very naughty thoughts.

If you know you are the one being watched, play it up for the camera! Get undressed in a room that you know is in his line of sight. You may be fulfilling his visual fantasy.

Scintillating Visuals

For some high-wattage optical thrills, porn stars suggest the following hot tactics to enhance visual foreplay. Don't forget to leave the lights on!

- Place a mirror in front of your couch or bed, then straddle your lover and start making out. This action, plus the bodacious view of your behind, will certainly amp up his visual pleasure.
- As you guide your lover to touch specific places on your body, leave an arm's-length distance between you. This way he can see both your body and your face as he arouses you.
- While in the 69 position, encourage your lover to lay his head on your inner thigh and take a peek at what you're doing to him.

With all this visual stimulation, the sexual tension will erupt into the hottest foreplay you've ever seen.

The Sounds of Sex

The decadent sounds of sex are powerful enough to send chills down your spine and get the juices flowing between your legs. The most expert connoisseurs, however, know that the sounds of sex are not confined to moans and groans alone. Flirtatious behavior and dirty talk can also get you and your lover revved up for getting down and dirty.

Not only do these sizzling sounds make your heart beat faster and your legs spread wider, but the creative effort you put into your sensual communication also expresses how much you care for your partner. You can build up your sexual repertoire while building a unique personal relationship with your lover that only the two of you share.

Down and Flirty

Just because your sexual relationship is private, that doesn't mean you can't express it in public. Actually, by publicly showcasing your playful side, you can begin seducing your lover long before physical foreplay begins. In porn scripts, the players always remember to keep the fire burning, even in social situations. So follow the steps below and discover some subtle, sexy ways to seduce your lover in the company of others.

- Never hesitate to tell your lover how sexy you find them. Verbal affirmation is just as important, and sometimes more important, than physical consummation.
- Sit close and touch each other in non-erogenous places like the arm, the leg, or the side, as conversation allows. Keep it natural and lighthearted, not chock-full of PDA.
- Turn it up a notch and touch yourself. Lightly caress your collarbone, play with your hair, or run your hands up and down your legs. He'll fantasize about touching those body parts himself during the entire night out!
- On a napkin, scribble "I'm not wearing any underwear," and then slide it to him. This tidbit of knowledge will drive your lover crazy and will keep him thinking of the sweet release planned for later on.
- Say playful things during conversations that only the two of you know the true meaning of.
- Banter back and forth about things that seem innocent on

the surface but that you and your partner find incredibility naughty.

• Flirt, flirt, and flirt, as if it is your first date and you already know that incredible sex is inevitable.

Green with Horny?

Porn stars know that a little jealousy can be a very good thing for your sex life. Flirting with others can show your partner your confidence, attractiveness, and spontaneity. It also gets your creative juices flowing for some dirty talk later that night. And that's always helpful for getting those juices below the belt to overflow.

One very important tip for this endeavor: Only flirt with random people you will never see again, like waiters, passersby, or that friendly stranger who held the door open for you—not friends, teachers, or your lover's family members. Not only would it seem disrespectful and way too close for sexual comfort to flirt with people close to you, it could also be very dangerous for your relationship.

Give It to Me, Baby

It's time to take your carnal conversation to the next level. Once you're alone with your lover, you'll need x-rated conversation to fire up x-rated moves. While we may poke fun at the dialogue in cheesy porn scenes outside the bedroom, we can definitely use those lines for inspiration inside the bedroom. For some reason, phrases that seem cheesy when your clothes are on can make your blood boil once they're off and your lover is between your legs.

How to Talk the Sexual Talk

Want to add some sexy sparks to your bedroom conversation but are shy about how to get those randy thoughts across? Follow the next steps and soon enough you'll be fanning his fire with porn-star passion.

- When sexy things pop into your head, just blurt them out. It feels freeing to express your innermost desires, and the more you do it, the more natural it will become. Plus, that type of honesty makes for the hottest comments.
- Just say "I love how you touch me." You'll see the steam rise!
- If you are too shy to come up with your own dirty script, you can always read someone else's. Bring some of your favorite erotica to bed and read it aloud to your lover.

Hitting the High Note

Get into a foxier frame of mind. Play a sensual CD during foreplay to get the momentum building. Depending upon the mood and the type of sex they're craving, porn stars list these as some all-time favorite songs to get busy to:

Making Sweet Love

- Let's Get It On—Marvin Gaye
- Unchained Melody—The Righteous Brothers
- 50 Candles—Boyz II Men
- That's the Way Love Goes—Janet Jackson
- No Ordinary Love—Sade

Fun Sex

- Can't Get Enough of Your Love, Babe—Barry White

- Cream—Prince
- Push It—Salt 'n' Pepa
- Dirrty—Christina Aguilera

Animalistic Sex
- Closer—Nine Inch Nails

Oral Sex
- Yummy, Yummy, Yummy (I've Got Love In My Tummy)
—Ohio Express
- Peaches and Cream—112

Fetishes
- Wicked Game—Chris Isaak

Rocking and Rolling
- Def Leppard—Pour Some Sugar on Me
- AC/DC—You Shook Me All Night Long

Ahhhh Baby!

There is nothing more sexually satisfying than hearing the natural gasps and groans of pleasure escaping our lips. These sounds not only give you the ability to communicate the enjoyment of touch without words, they also can prolong foreplay by encouraging your lover to

> Do some light role-playing to build up the sexual anticipation between you and your lover. Jokingly take on another couple's style and talk the way they would. Once you get into bed, stay in character and verbally seduce each other. No costumes required!

continue his pleasure-causing actions. Plus, the thought that you have no control over your outcries makes your partner aware that you are in the same sexual moment with him.

Porn stars want you to rise up from whatever social restrictions cause you to silence your satisfaction. Remember, the sounds of sex are natural music to our ears. Never be shy about uninhibitedly expressing your pleasure in the throes of passion.

> Foreplay not only benefits the emotional connection a couple can feel as they are making love, it also can aid with some other technical aspects of intercourse. Foreplay literally helps get your juices flowing, and all that natural lube aids deeper penetration once you do have sex. Also, the longer the foreplay, the more heightened the sexual anticipation and the stronger your orgasms. So no matter how you approach it, you can't go wrong with some pleasurable attention to detail.

BON APPETIT

Let your lover know that he is your favorite meal. Savor every inch of his skin by exploring it with your lips and your tongue. Use your hunger for sex as the ultimate foreplay technique, and sample each part of his body as an appetizer for what is sure to come. Exploring your partner's taste prolongs the anticipation of sweet release, so eat to your heart's content.

> Enjoy a light appetizer! Give your lover a passionate kiss before work or while out in public. This will build the sexual tension between you that will explode into satisfaction later on.

Ultimate Kisses

Kissing is the spark that ignites my inner furnace, and without it I might as well masturbate.

—Nina Hartley

Candlelight Kissing

Kissing is the ultimate expression of sexual appetite. Unfortunately, it also is often the first element of foreplay to be overlooked. A couple can begin a romance entangled in passionate, earth shattering lip-locks that last for hours, but slowly regress into tight-lipped pecks that are over in seconds once familiarity sets in. Too often we forget that a simple deep kiss can make our knees weak and our pussies tremble.

So do a little mouth-to-mouth resuscitation on your kissing skills and revive them by reinstating some porn-star passion.

THE Kiss

Cradle your lover's face in your hands and kiss him gently. Then lean him against a wall or a door, raise his hands above his head and start kissing more deeply. Then nuzzle your face into his neck and kiss him sweetly there while running your hands up and down his body. Return to his face for a kiss. Take his face into your hands and kiss him deeply again. You will feel his body melt into yours.

The French Kiss

At times, this technique is not executed in the intended manner. Many people insert their entire tongue into their partner's mouth. The real way to French kiss is to use only the tip of the tongue. Start kissing and insert the tip of your tongue into your partner's mouth. Circle his tongue with yours. Pull back and play with your lover's lips. Repeat.

> Take the foreplay reins. Kiss him seductively, then pull away and say "If you want more you better come and get it!"

Sweet Kissing

While passionate kisses generate heat, sweet kisses keep the fire burning. Kissing these areas is sensual in nature, not sexual, and can express the caring feelings you have for your partner:

> The ultimate sweet kiss is named "The Wrist Kiss," but it'll be sure to make your lover weak in the knees. Hold your lips against the wrist of your lover until you can feel his pulse with your lips. Look into his eyes the entire time. Then kiss him passionately on the lips, holding his face within your hands. Then return to kiss his wrist. See how much faster his pulse beats the second time around.

- Forehead
- Cheeks
- Top of Head
- Chest
- Shoulders
- Ears

Remember, kissing is not the only way you can taste your lover's scrumptious skin. Suck his earlobes, toes, fingers, and any other areas you deem delicious! The feeling of your mouth around his fingers will make him think of your mouth around other appendages.

The Body Trail

Often lovers get stuck kissing and sucking the same areas, then jumping right to penetration. The key to ending this boring routine is to avoid the expected hot spots and explore your lover's entire body. This also communicates the idea that making love with your partner is not all about your own sexual gratification but is about mutual sensual satisfaction.

To heighten the overall sexual experience, kiss your partner's body all over and stay away from genital stimulation for as long as possible. Try tasting these less-visited places of pleasure, which are chock-full of nerve endings, and see how quickly your lover begs you to quench his thirst for more:

- Nipples
- Temples
- Eyelids
- Hollow of throat
- Behind earlobes
- The angle where your neck meets your shoulder

For some below-the-belt kisses that will cheer you both up, try the following scandalous spots:

- Inner Thighs
- Buttock
- Back of Knees

When you just can't take it anymore, start kissing these hot-hotter-hottest spots:

Specifically for Him

- **The H-Spot: His corona.** Run your tongue around the bottom edge of his penis head, where the head meets the shaft. It'll make him salivate for more.
- **The R-Spot: His raphe.** The very visible line running along the center of his scrotum is called a "raphe." Keep the lights on and lick between the lines!
- **The P-Spot: His perineum.** The area between the anus and the base of the scrotum is called the "perineum." Rich in

nerve endings, this area is often overlooked by women. Be the first one to sample this area of skin and rock his world!

Specifically for Her

- **The C-Spot: Her clitoris.** Lick slowly up one side and down the other, and you'll have her begging for more.
- **The G-Spot:** If you insert your finger into her vagina and make a "come hither" movement, you'll feel a spongy spot. This is the famous G-spot, and just touching it alone can produce orgasms in many women.

> He has a G-spot too! You can reach it two ways, either by pressing his perineum with your thumb or by inserting a finger into his anus and making a "come hither" movement. It's about time you were able to make him come merely by lifting a finger!

- **The U-Spot: Her urethra.** This is the tiny area of tissue above her vagina opening. Stimulate this area if her clitoris is too sensitive for immediate touch following orgasm.

Flavorful Foreplay

Want to bring your taste buds into the bedroom? Incorporate some tasty items into your sex play, like edible body paint, flavored condoms, honey dust, and edible panties. The tasty possibilities are endless!

Or pour some of these tasty substances onto your

> Don't let your mouth have all the fun. While in a steamy make-out session, remember to use your hands to heighten the experience. Caress and stroke each other's bodies while in lip-lock, and let the petting intensify as the kisses get steamier.

favorite parts of your lover. They'll be sure to make your mouth water!

- Chocolate
- Whipped Cream
- Champagne
- Honey
- Whiskey

SENSUOUS SCENTS

Scent has the power to bring back fond memories from our unconscious. Sunscreen may remind us of childhood summers, funnel cakes may bring us back to youthful days at a carnival, and the smell of a particular soap may remind us of a tantalizing tryst in the bathtub.

While some don't see scent as a key element of foreplay, porn stars know that with a little creativity, this intoxicating sense can compete with the best of them to get your juices flowing. Try using distinctive scents during your next randy romp so that when you smell them again, it will stir up those erotic memories. The following tips will help you incorporate scent into your sexual repertoire.

- Lather each other's bodies with a light scented soap in the shower, in anticipation of a long sweaty sex session afterward.
- Sprinkle flower petals on the bed—not just for the romance factor, but also for the scent. As your bodies crush the petals during deeper petting foreplay, the fragrance will fill the room.
- Rub down each other's bodies with scented lotion after body-awakening morning sex.
- Light some scented candles next time you have dinner, then be sure to have some sweet and delicious sex for dessert.

- Remember the simple fact that your lover's cologne makes you weak in the knees.

A Fragrance for Every Mood

Fragrances are powerful enough to change someone's mood instantly. So what scintillating scents do porn stars suggest using when you want your lover to switch gears from "not now" to "let's get it on"? Next time you want to hit the sheets for some slow burning love, use the following scents in candles and oils:

Citrus: This scent increases energy and creativity, which always makes for the best kind of lovemaking!

Lavender: After a long day of work, this scent inspires relaxation and allows you to get your happy hour even after you and your lover have clocked out.

Pine and Mint: These fragrances can raise anyone's spirits (and that kind of invigoration will make a certain someone stand at attention!).

Jasmine/Gardenia/Sandalwood/Rose: These scents generate warmth and feelings of romance. Use these when you want some sweet lovemaking.

Cinnamon: Any spicy scent will inspire your lover to make things hot.

And for the ultimate scent stimulation…

The Scandalous Back Massage

Use scented oils and create some sizzling memories with these seductive massages.

For Him

Sit on his ass while naked and begin massaging scented oils into his bare back. As you pay attention to his upper back and forearms, be sure to lean forward so he can feel your naked nipples and breasts on his skin. Rub your nipples down his back as you use your hands the massage the rest of this area.

Bonus: Have your lover reach his arms behind his back and play with your clit as you give him a massage. The attention he gives you will remind you that he's in this for you as well.

For Her

Sit on her ass while naked and begin massaging scented oils into her bare back. Caress her sides and lavishly kiss up her spine for as long as she can take it. When you feel she is wet and ready, slip inside her for some doggy-style action.

TANTALIZING TOUCH

And speaking of seductive massages, it's time to get down on your knees, ignite the fire, and begin worshipping your lover's luscious body. Don't leave one spot unexplored or one curvaceous crevice untouched. The act of touch—caressing, massaging, tickling, petting—can bring lovers closer together on a sensual level. Plus, the fine attention to delicious detail helps rev up our rockets for one serious blastoff.

Porn stars know that sensual skin-to-skin contact is essential to good sex and is the secret to happiness itself. Naturally they have tips for giving and receiving this type of carnal worship.

Non-Sexual Healing

Porn stars know how important sex is to any healthy relationship. But even they know you have to balance the need for good old-fashioned fucking and the need for comfort. Non-sexual caresses let your lover know you care enough to put his comfort before your sexual needs. These tender, arousing ways of touching soothe the savage breast, but often lead to more:

- Massaging your lover's scalp. Stroke his forehead, from the center to the temples. Press lightly on his temples, and then release. This relieves any tension or strain that may have had your partner feeling not-in-the-mood.
- Hold hands. Caress the back of your lover's hand with your thumb. This move mimics how you may touch other areas of his body.
- Cuddle. It's sensual and soothing, and the perfect segue into something deeper.
- Lightly caress your partner's wrist, resting your thumb on his pulse. If he thinks his heart is beating now, wait until you're done with him!

Deep Petting

Now you're ready to delve into some deeper, can't-wait-to-get-it-on touches. While caressing has always been a precursor to sex, here are some porn-star tips for making it as memorable as the lovemaking itself.

The Sexual Touch

Body

- Using the pads of your fingers, lightly rack your hands up and down your lover's body.
- Run your fingers from one erogenous zone to another. Start slowly and apply more pressure as you go along. The variations in touch will have your lover hungering for more. Make sure to linger in the genital area.
- Grab and squeeze your lover's butt, and ask him to squeeze yours at the same time. You'll not only feel connected with this move, you can also draw each other's bodies closer to one another.

Nipples

- Just like sex itself, this is a his-and-hers pleasure. Use your thumbs to press the nipples in gently, then rub around them for a few seconds.
- You also can brush your fingers lightly across aroused nipples for a teasing sensation.
- For deeper foreplay, add some oral play. Lightly kiss your lover's nipples. Nibble them, suck them gently, and run your tongue back and forth across them.
- Blow lightly over your partner's nipples. You'll see them stand at attention!

Chest

- There are pleasure points on your lover's chest that, when stimulated, send chills up and down his body. These are found on either side of the breastbone, at approximately nipple level, halfway between the nipples and the center of the sternum. Touch this area lightly with your finger for a few seconds and you'll see spine-tingling results.

Breasts

• Hand this book over to your lover so he can indulge in these randy tips.

• When you want to tantalize a woman with touch, do not squeeze her breasts or pinch her nipples.

• Stroke and massage them with the palms of your hands.

• Run your hands up and down the sides; caress them simultaneously, push them together, and lavish them with attention.

> Sizzling foreplay is all about multi-tasking. Don't just stimulate one hot zone at a time. While you are lavishing his nipples with attention, caress his butt as well. It will feel like you are making love to his entire body.

Masturbation Magic

All this rubbing, licking, and feather-light touching can make one yearn for deeper petting. While masturbation is usually seen as a solo endeavor, porn stars know that thinking outside the box is what makes foreplay fantastic. They realize that masturbating in front of each other not only educates you on how your partner gets his or her juices flowing, it also can bring you closer to each other emotionally. Besides, seeing your partner touching himself is extremely hot to watch!

The Ultimate Foreplay Lesson

Mutual masturbation can be as much as a learning tool as it is a turn-on. Masturbate side-by-side while kissing and caressing each other. Pay attention to what he may be doing to himself when the kisses get deeper. You'll see that those are the moves he craves from you, and vice versa.

You can also masturbate each other in this fashion. Use one hand to pleasure your lover while using the other to show him exactly how to masturbate you. He'll learn from hands-on experience what turns you on, turns you off, and turns your heat up. Now that kind of knowledge definitely is power!

For a more heightened experience, lie side by side as close you can without touching and masturbate yourselves with your eyes closed. Your senses of smell and hearing will kick in. You may not be able to see what makes your lover's breath quicken, but you may discover what sighs are more urgent than others. This unique lesson will bring you closer to understanding your lover's sexual needs.

As an added bonus, you may feel more comfortable touching yourself during sex now that you have done so in front of your partner. Now you can heighten your own sexual experience by rubbing your clit or your breasts next time you're getting down-and-dirty. Not only will this bring you closer to orgasm, but seeing that you are a confident sex kitten will also drive your lover crazy with passion.

And remember, never ever feel that masturbation is shameful. It allows for self-awareness and teaches our lovers how to shower us with heavenly bliss. There is no sin in that.

> Remember, all individuals are turned on by different touches, strokes, and caresses. To connect sexually with your lover and give him everything he desires in bed, spend extended amounts of time seducing each other. The results are well worth the effort.

Virgin Passion

Remember those youthful days when sex was yet to be discovered and even the idea of almost going all the way was thrilling and forbidden? All that fondling and sexual tension was enough to get your panties in a bunch!

Nowadays your pants come off before your panties even have a chance to get wet. There was something to be said for your sexual past and holding off until the last possible second before penetration. Seduction was the main event, and you could never get enough.

It's time to go back to basics, spark some sexy memories, and bump and grind like it was prom night.

Bump and Grind

Stay fully dressed during this tantalizing technique. Kiss and caress each other through your clothes until you can't stand it any longer. Begin bumping up against your lover on the upstroke and grinding down on his package on the downstroke. Wrap your leg around his waist, or rest your foot on a step for balance. But in order to heighten the sweet anticipation, don't lie down.

Dry Sex

This was the loving you craved before you discovered the spectacle of sex. Both you and your partner may remove all your clothing except for your underwear. Focus your attention on all the delicious skin above the waist until you're dying for some deeper petting. Then tease and tantalize each other through your underthings with your tongues and hands. As your hearts race, climb into an intercourse position and mimic the moves of making love. You'll discover how easy it is to reach orgasm without penetration!

> The mind is the primary sex organ. You need to be mentally stimulated to the fullest in order to be fully aroused for sex. Make sure all your senses are erotically indulged so that when penetration does occur, you're all wet and raring to go!

See It to Believe It!

Our porn vixens list their favorite educational videos on how to always keep your foreplay hot and steamy:

Joy of Erotic Massage—Sinclair Intimacy Institute, 2001, 60 minutes

Nina Hartley's Guide to Seduction—Adam and Eve Productions, 1997, 120 minutes

Talk To Me Baby: A Lover's Guide to Dirty Talk and Role Play—SIR Video, 2003, 60 minutes

The Secrets of Self-Pleasuring and Mutual Masturbation—Sinclair Intimacy Institute, 1999, 35 minutes

Bonus Tip: Always remember: Seductive foreplay doesn't end when fornication begins. During sex, continue to lavish your lover's body as you ravish it.

Going Down to Pleasure Town

HOW TO FOLLOW THE MAP TO THE MOST DELICIOUS ORAL SEX YOUR MOUTH HAS EVER TASTED

> If you have the ambition to suck cock like a porn star, you'll eventually learn how, but in the meantime you can both enjoy a process of discovery that need never be less than pleasant in any way.
>
> —Nina Hartley

Porn stars know not only how sensual oral sex looks on the silver screen, they also know how incredibly good it is when done correctly. The good news is, it's easy to learn the secrets of using your tongue to give tantalizing pleasure between the sheets.

Porn actors know, too, that there is nothing degrading about kneeling in front of your lover to focus on his pleasure. Actually, there is an erotic power to be found in being able to use your mouth alone to bring your lover over the edge. It gives you full control of his body, and it gets you all wet knowing you're making his juices overflow.

So if you're serious about moving toward becoming fully sexually satisfied, drop to your knees.

HIS CUP RUNNETH OVER

The porn industry put blowjobs on the map in a major way with a little movie named *Deep Throat*. Since then, men of all types have raised oral sex to the level of a living and breathing necessity.

While some of us are lucky enough to get a whole banana down our throats before our gag reflex kicks in, however, others have to learn the trade secrets of sucking cock.

So whether it's an appetizer or the main course for you, here are some tips for stroking, licking, and sucking cock with a passion.

Blowjob Basics

Get down to the basics while you're down on your knees.

- Kiss and lick his inner thighs but don't touch his penis. The anticipation will drive him crazy.
- Just when you think he can't take it anymore, begin gently stroking up and down the shaft of his penis. Moisten your hands with oil and use both hands to twist in opposite directions as you slide up and down his shaft.
- Wet your lips and then run your tongue around the tip of his cock, to moisten it.
- With one hand, hold the base of his penis and with the other make a circle with your thumb and forefinger around the shaft, and slide that up and down while you suck him. This prevents him from going farther into your mouth

than you'd like while giving him the feeling of friction on his entire cock.

- Begin licking and sucking his head while you stroke him with a twisting motion with the other hand.
- Swirl your tongue around the tip of his cock as if licking an ice-cream cone. Then alternate with longer tongue strokes up and down the shaft.
- Take as much of his penis as you can into your entire mouth, then suck as you pull him out. Repeat if possible.
- If you're feeling daring, rub his penis between your breasts as you keep your head down. Lick the tip every time it comes up between your breasts.
- Use your tongue to lick the corona while continuing to stroke him with your other hand. Suck the head of his cock.
- Take breaks between all that licking and sucking. Take him out of your mouth and stroke him as you make eye contact.
- Don't neglect his other body parts. Grab his butt firmly or run your fingers up and down his chest while you're getting busy on his member.
- Repeat any steps that cause him to moan with pleasure.
- Start slow and sensually. But be prepared to move quicker closer to his orgasm. A large amount of friction is needed for him to blast off.
- Make eye contact.
- As he cums, gently apply pressure to his perineum with your thumb.

Ask any man what his blowjob basic is and he'll tell you that eye contact is key. Show him the confident porn-star goddess you are, and make eye contact as you blow him over the edge.

Small Tips for a Huge Happy Ending

- Hum while his cock is in your mouth. The vibrations will drive him crazy.
- Don't neglect the boys. Rub, suck, and lick his testicles for added sensation.
- Play with yourself while he's in your mouth. The visual alone is smoking hot and will remind him that this is for both of you.
- Grab a few ice cubes and keep them beside the bed. Place one in your mouth while you go down on him. The cold sensation combined with the warmth of your mouth will drive him crazy. Brushing your teeth with minty toothpaste before you go down on him will have the same effect!
- Lick his shaft like it was an ice-cream cone. Suck it like it was your favorite hard candy (who are we kidding?—it is!)

> **Location, Location, Location**
> Every porn star knows you don't always have to kneel in front of your lover to give him a mind-blowing blowjob. Next time your mouth is craving some candy, lie down on the couch as he straddles your mouth. He can use the cushions to hang on.

Some Tantalizing Techniques

All porn stars can tell you that getting the basics down can lead to a blowjob he'll never forget. However, they also have some scandalous techniques in their closets that'll make you the lover he never forgets.

The Bark in Your Bite

When you begin going down on your lover, put his cock into your mouth before he hardens. Start sucking and licking until he swells to the point where he no longer fits. As you wrap your lips around his shaft and start pulling him out, bite gently and slowly onto his head until you feel a delicious quiver. Release quickly and then take him into your mouth again.

The Power of the Gag Reflex

If your lover is craving some deep sucking and you want to give it to him, Nina Hartley suggests that a small gag reflex on your part might actually get his juices pumping. The slight involuntary contraction of your throat muscles around his cock is similar to the sensation of an orgasm. If you can tolerate three or four almost-gags in a row, he'll be so hot he won't even notice when you return to focusing solely on the tip of his cock.

The Nerve of Him

Many women shy away from oral sex because they fear their gag reflex will kick in, their libido will give out, and their lover will be disappointed. However, many porn stars know the truth. The most responsive parts of a man's member are the tip and along the first quarter of the shaft because these contain the largest number of nerve endings. So you don't need to be Deep Throat to satisfy him. You can still rock his world orally without losing your lunch.

The Wake-Up Call

Next time you wake up in a frisky mood and your lover is still asleep, press your face against the bulb of his cock. Lift up his penis and spread his balls apart, and then plant a warm deep kiss on the space between. Stroke the entire full length of his cock with both your hands. Then put him entirely in your mouth and suck upward. Release your mouth when you come to the tip. It'll be the sexiest wake-up call he's ever had.

> If your lover happens not to be circumcised, there are some specific tricks your tongue can do to bring him to a frenzy. Pull the foreskin over the head of his penis and squeeze it together. Gently lick, nibble, suck, and explore the folds of that delicious skin.

To Spit or to Swallow

It is a man-law that your lover must tell you when he is about to cum when you're working on his package. This allows you to decide if you want to swallow his love juices, spit them out after he cums, or remove your mouth entirely and have him cum somewhere else on your delicious body. Always discuss these options before you begin, not only to avoid confusion but also to heighten the sexual anticipation.

- If you do decide to swallow but are still getting used to his taste, position yourself so that his cum will shoot straight down your throat. Lie on your back with your head off the bed and have him straddle your face. This way your mouth and throat form a direct line for his cum to go down smoothly. No taste buds need be involved.

- Another hot technique: When he is near ejaculation, take his pelvis in both hands and thrust him toward you so he goes deeper into your mouth. Then swallow.

Swallowing is definitely worth the extra credit. It makes your lover feel totally accepted and loved when you swallow his juices. He'll be sure to pay you back for this treat with some extra loving of his own.

However, if you opt instead for that classic porn move, the cum shot, here are some traditional places to have him explode:

- Stomach
- Breasts
- Cheeks
- Lips

> Next time you're feeling a little adventurous when you're on a road trip with your lover, give him a little treat. While he is driving, pull out his cock and lick and suck your way to a blissful destination. Just be sure he's able to concentrate on the road, since road head can be a very distracting way to travel to Pleasuretown.

Note: Avoid eyes. No matter how many times you may have seen it in porn movies, it is not safe or pleasant for the receiving partner.

CUNNING CUNNILINGUS SKILL

It has been reported that many women in their twenties are less assertive about getting their oral needs met than older women. It's time for sex stars around the world to unite and share the secrets of orally getting your rocks off. These pros know that it isn't always easy to ask your lover for the oral action you're craving. They suggest discussing these needs with your lover by way of some naughty pillow talk. He'll be sure to listen.

Join the revolution! Here are some racy requests to make next time he's on his knees.

- Request that he write the alphabet on your vulva with his

tongue. He should tease the entire area and leave your clit for last.

- Ask him to make humming sounds as he licks and kisses your clit—the vibrations will send you over the edge.

- As you are cumming, ask him to lick you in slow, even strokes. Once your orgasm subsides, have him begin light, rapid flicks of his tongue once again.

> Men are generally happy to listen to any suggestions their lover gives them that will heighten her pleasure. Stop being shy about your needs. That boy is craving direction! A naughty request alone will bring him to his knees.

The Map to Pleasure Town

We know you are a confident, secure, and adventurous woman. You like to take what is yours by the balls instead of dancing around it. Map out the directions to your pleasure town by having your lover read the following steps.

- Tease and tantalize her body before diving right onto her genitals. Make sure she is fully aroused before your tongue even touches her clitoris.

- While kissing her, place your hand over her vulva and squeeze. The sensation of the heel of your hand moving her clit into your fingers is spine tingling.

- Once you've touched her to the point where she needs some deeper petting, it's time to move down south. Gently part her labia with your tongue. Lick the delicious tissue along the sides and above and below her clitoris with long strokes of your tongue.

- Vary tongue strokes to see which ones are the most effective. She'll moan when you get it right.

- While you are stroking her labia with your hands, you can gently bite her inner thighs. Then kiss all the way back to her clitoral area.
- Place your lips around her clitoris. Hold them in a kissing position as you gently suck. You can alternate this sucking with licking the surrounding area and light licks directly on her clitoris.
- As she is near orgasm, cover her clitoral area with your entire mouth. Suck the surrounding area, and with your hands, tease her nipples and stroke her inner thighs.
- Do not move your mouth until she has reached orgasm. Once she hits the point of no return and you feel her orgasm in your mouth, it will have paid to have been patient and determined.

> Never imitate the exaggerated tongue flicks seen in porn movies. While they may look dazzling on screen, smaller, gentler licks are the ones that send a woman over the edge.

Some Tantalizing Techniques

Her body is a temple, so worship and ravish her. Here are some scandalous skills to learn.

The Flame

Pretend that the tip of your tongue is a candle flame and that flame is flickering in the wind. Move your tongue rapidly over her pussy, above and below her clit, and across her vulva the way a flame would flicker in the wind. Use the tip of your tongue and flick back and forth only along the clitoral shaft. As she is coming to orgasm, flick back and forth along the entire top of the clitoris.

This can be too much direct stimulation for some women. Find out if your lover likes direct contact. If not, have her keep her panties on while you do this. The indirect stimulation may be what she needs, and the naughty image will be sure to keep you fully engaged.

No, the Pleasure Is All Mine

Hold the tip of your tongue against her clitoris and move your head back and forth as if you were saying "no, no, no." You'll be sure to make her scream "yes, yes, yes!"

Foot Fetish

While she is on her back, tilt her so that the arch of one foot is on the bed. Rub your cock against this arch while you're eating her out. Not only will it feel better than rumpled sheets against your penis, but also, feet are full of nerve endings and she'll love the contact. Besides, enacting this racy porn move is sexy in and of itself.

The Twofer

As you are using your tongue to bring her over the edge during orgasm, stimulate her G-Spot with your fingers at the same time. It will feel like her orgasm is coming from both places and will resound throughout her entire vagina.

THE POWER OF 69

While the mouth-watering 69 position is all about simultaneous

Location, Location, Location
Have him worship you in the best way possible; on his knees. Have him kneel down in the shower as you wrap your legs around his shoulders.

oral stimulation, there is also something hot about taking your turn.

- When your lover is flicking and licking away, you can pause on your licking and sucking and keep his penis still in your mouth. This allows you to concentrate on the pleasure and your hot rapid breaths on his member will keep him hard as you get your rocks off. When you feel the waves of pleasure approaching, switch your concentration onto him. This will increase endurance and heighten pleasure.
- While you're using all your newfound techniques and going to town on your lover's cock, have him keep still and rest his mouth on your vulva. His hot rapid breaths will have the same effects on you as yours do on him. When you feel he's ready for blastoff, stop and have the focus return back to you.

HAND JOB HEAVEN

Pleasure Him Silly

Never underestimate the power of the hand job. Many women skip this enticing technique because they think this is something their lover can do for himself and that their lover desires something *more* from them besides touch. However, porn stars know the truth and can tell you how to use your hands to give your lover *more* than his own hands could ever give.

- First, have some lube handy. You may start dry, but as you get into it, some type of lube (or your saliva) will allow you to pull off the more intense moves that send him over the edge.

- Interlace your fingers and clasp them snugly over his shaft. Move them up and down in a twisting motion. You can vary the movement by eliminating the twist.
- Now that his penis is hard, focus solely on the tip. Gently grasp and release your hands around the bottom of the shaft and move up slowly at about one second intervals. Stop at the corona (the rim where the shaft meets the head) and feel him quiver in your hands.
- Repeat these twisting and contracting strokes until he is ready to blast off. During the grand finale, hold him firmly with both hands and contract them in time with his spasms.
- If this doesn't get his rocks off, you can hold his penis like a joystick and rub his shaft up and down, keeping his penis between your palms. You may start slowly, but you will need to increase speed and pressure as he reaches orgasm.
- As he finishes, run your thumb from the base of the underside of his shaft up to the head. That last touch will give him goose bumps.

Send Her to the Moon

Let's not forget about our own pleasure. Hand this book over to your lover and let him learn all about the way his hands can bring you over the edge.

- Start with caressing her inner thighs, using your palms in upward strokes. Work your way to her genitals in the same manner. Part her lips gently and stroke her inner labia.
- Some women like their clitoris directly stroked. If she does, take it between your thumb and forefinger and gently rotate. If she doesn't, massage the entire area.

- Make a V shape with your fingers and hold it around her clitoris. Press down lightly and then pull back. Repeat. This rocking motion can bring her to orgasm. If not, you can alternate the circular massage around her clitoris, the rotating move, and the V technique until she does.

See It to Believe It!

Watch the following educational videos to see exactly what these sex kittens mean when they say "hard-on." Learning has never been so much fun!

Better Oral Sex Techniques—Pacific Media Entertainment, 1997, 60 minutes

Complete Guide to Oral Lovemaking—Pacific Media Entertainment, 1997, 60 minutes

Nina Hartley's Advanced Guide to Oral Sex—Nina Hartley, 1998, 45 minutes

Bonus Tip: Always remember: Enthusiasm is more important than technique. Eagerness to please your lover will always be reciprocated.

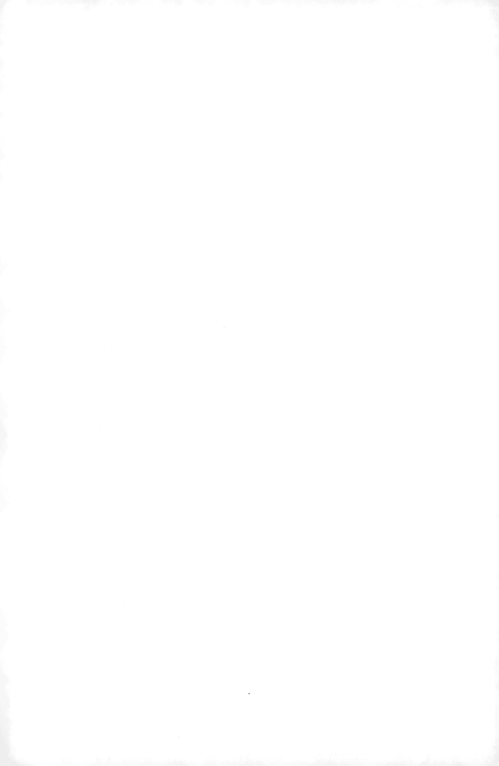

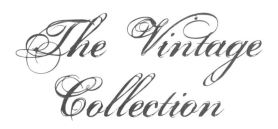

The Vintage Collection

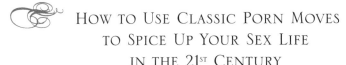

HOW TO USE CLASSIC PORN MOVES TO SPICE UP YOUR SEX LIFE IN THE 21ST CENTURY

Sex is an emotion in motion.

—Mae West

There are some images that just scream (and moan) "porn" when they pop into our heads. Some of these, however, are acrobatic endeavors that may look spectacular on screen but don't actually feel spectacular between the sheets. Besides, exotic positions are always performed by porn pros. Attempting to replicate some of them in your own home may produce more "ouches" than "ahhs."

Luckily, there are some classic positions and techniques that have great pizzazz *and* make sparks fly. And of course porn stars have tips on how to make these carnal classics even steamier! Now you'll be able to put a naughty twist on some old favorites, and ignite serious fireworks with new ones.

TRIED AND TRUE TRADITIONAL POSITIONS
The simplest of sexual positions can be the hottest. The

missionary position is uncomplicated. Spooning is easy. Getting it on in traditional positions is seamless and effortless, and allows lovers to focus on sensations, sensuality, and the intensity of the fire they're creating. Plus, the simplicity of these positions often can bring you back to your first days of knocking boots and remind you how the spark was lit in the first place.

A Mission into the Wild—Missionary Position

Throw caution to the wind and throw away the belief that the missionary position is purely puritanical. Actually, with the right amount of passion, this act can be every bit as adventurous as you are!

Assume the Position:

After some sensual foreplay, lie on your back and have your lover kneel between your legs and press his cock firmly against your pussy. Since you'll be wet and raring to go from all your pre-nooky pleasure, he'll be able to sink into you easily. Have him slide all the way in and rest his full weight on you.

The Ample Advantages

- This position promotes intense intimacy, because you can easily hug, kiss, look into each other's eyes, and rub every inch of each other's bodies. Plus, there is a sensual primal pleasure to be found in being pinned down and deeply penetrated.
- This position also allows for the best views! You can watch your lover's cock go in and out, giving you some hot carnal images to stoke your fire. And if he catches you sneaking a peek it'll just spike his lust even more.

Titillating Techniques

- Let your lover know that the relentless, in-and-out, hammering motion typical of many porn films is unacceptable! Have him grind against you in an up-and-down motion instead. Ask him to push his weight upward while he pushes inward, to stimulate your clit, and to drop down when he slides out, to hit your G-spot.
- Place a small pillow under your butt. This way, when your lover enters you, your vaginal canal is at a better angle to accommodate his cock, which translates into deeper penetration and more access to your G-spot. Another way to get these results: put your legs on his shoulders.
- Reach simultaneous orgasm in this purrfect position. The CAT (Coital Alignment Technique) allows for delicious pressure on your clitoris at the same time he's getting some frisky friction on the base of his cock. Lie on your back and have your lover lie on top of you so that his pelvis is higher than your clitoris. Wrap your legs around his thighs and rest your ankles on his calves. Move only your pelvises in a slow, steady rhythm without ever speeding up or slowing down. Push upward on the upstroke and have your partner push downward on the down stroke. Repeat until you both explode. Despite the leisurely nature of this position, you'll soon discover that slow-and-steady wins the race!

Fight the theory that the missionary position is demure and dainty by fucking back. Display how ravenous you are by meeting all his thrusts with full-force thrusts of your own, to achieve deliciously deep penetration, or simply ask him to stay still as you fuck him from underneath his weight.

Fork Me Baby—Spooning

Play sweet 'n' sexy in this position. Next time you're craving a little "forking," ask your lover to take you gently from behind. It'll be a cuddling session he'll never forget!

Assume the Position:

Lie on your side with your lover behind you. Angle your butt so it is right up against him and have him enter you from behind as he puts one leg between yours. While it is a little more difficult to achieve friction in this position, the intimacy level makes the effort worth the reward in the end.

The Ample Advantages

- This position is perfect for when you're both very tired but also very horny. Execution is effortless and the sensations are steamy!
- Three words: Full body contact!
- Your lover can easily caress your hair and has great access to your neck and breasts. Plus you both have great access to your clit!

Titillating Techniques

- Have your lover increase the depth of his thrusts by pushing and pulling your shoulders to and from him. The feeling of being held by the shoulders and pulled back into a rigid cock is deeply satisfying. Or, for the same effect, simply use your bodies as leverage against each other.
- Spice up his morning by rubbing your ass against his cock to wake him up, and stay in this position as he takes you then and there. Who needs coffee with this kind of sex rush?!

Giddy-Up Cowgirl—Woman on Top

Get ready for some riding lessons! Mount your lover and get yours the way you want it.

Assume the Position:

In this versatile and powerful position, you can mount your lover and either rest your knees on either side of his chest, keep your legs alongside his and balance yourself with your hands, or sit upright and have both hands free.

The Ample Advantages

- This position is traditionally a female favorite, not only because the woman has complete control, but also because it normally guarantees that she orgasms. With all that clit stimulation, it's hard not to!
- It's very sexually liberating since you have the freedom to meet all your own sexual needs, from controlling the depth and speed of thrusting to being able to stroke your own clit during intercourse for added stimulation.
- He loves it because he gets a great view of your entire exposed body and has excellent access to all your erogenous zones. He'll be sure to lavish and ravish your face, neck, breasts, torso, and clit with attention.

Titillating Techniques

- Move in circular movements instead of the up-and-down of normal thrusting. If you still crave the in-and-out feeling, thrust downward on the downward curve of the circle and thrust upward on the upward curve of the circle. Lean slightly forward so there is constant clitoral stimulation.

- Instead of mounting your lover with him lying down, prop him up in a comfy chair or against the headboard. This way you can just sit atop him, your hips have more freedom to move, and his mouth is right at nipple level! The combination of his swirling cock and your clit rubbing against his abdomen will ignite a blazing blastoff.

- Give your lover the ultimate lap dance. Tell him to sit in a chair, ask him to follow erotic orders, and inform him that he can look but he may not touch. Start with a sexy striptease and then mount him and insert his cock in your pussy. (Then let him know he can touch all he wants!)

QUIVERING QUICKIES

In this fast-paced world of 8 a.m. meetings, super-sized meals, and sixty-hour work weeks, career couples are more likely to save sex for the weekends. Porn stars ask, Why would you go five whole days without primal pleasure? Here are some quick ideas for satisfying quickies that can end your weekday abstinence dilemma.

- Mount your lover as he is sitting innocently watching television. Quickly take off both of your clothes. The sight and surprise of it all should give him at least a semi-erection. Insert this inside of you as you ride him up and down. Keep your legs as open as possible so that when you're thrusting, your clitoris is stimulated by the underside of his cock. He'll quickly get hard and you'll both quickly cum—the perfect quickie equation.

- Start on a hot note. Read some erotica, watch some porn, or masturbate in the bathroom, whatever it takes to be all revved up when you tackle your man for a quickie.

- Fantasize. Everyone has a kinky little fantasy in their closet. Bring it out during a quickie and use it to get highly aroused.

> Don't let puritanical beliefs or politics hold you back. The more you can relax and accept the pleasure riveting through your body, the more energy you can focus on rocking your lover's world!

PORNOGRAPHIC POSITIONS

Some days you're going to want it harder, deeper, and a little more complicated. So indulge in some of the more pornographic positions, including Doggy Style and Reverse Cowgirl. These positions are porn clichés for a randy reason—they just feel so good! They involve a little more flexibility and balance, but all the effort and concentration pays off in great penetration and fantastic friction!

Give Me a Bone—Doggy Style

It's passionate, primal, and the best position for deep penetration. Rediscover your inner sex kitten!

Assume the Position:

Get on all fours and kneel in front of your partner. Have him enter you from behind. You actually can control the depth of penetration by either staying on your knees or lowering your chest to the bed and raising your ass.

The Ample Advantages

- Anatomically speaking, this sexual position is the ideal fit for males and females. Plus, there is something raw and animalistic about being taken from behind. The alignment alone can awaken the primitive lust in both of you!

- This position allows for deeper penetration and therefore better G-spot stimulation.
- It's very sexy to forgo face-to-face intimacy in this position. You can release all inhibitions and lose yourself in pleasure.
- For added stimulation, rub your own clit or introduce a vibrator into the mix.
- You get an added jolt of pleasure when his balls slap against your clit.
- The visuals are very randy! He gets to revel in the splendor of your butt and you get a great view of his cock sliding in and out of you!

Titillating Techniques

- Ask him to combine his deep thrusts with some hair pulling and neck biting. The dual sensations will drive you doubly crazy!
- Have your lover firmly spread your ass cheeks while in this position. The opening of your derrière will give him a great visual treat, and the sensation will feel really good for you too!
- Instead of staying on all fours, lie on your stomach in a "collapsed doggy" position and have your partner enter you from behind. Keep your legs straight behind you

> For some added kink, have your lover use a gloved, lubed-up thumb to stimulate your anus for some soaring sensations.

and have his legs lie outside yours. Then you can easily fuck him by demanding he stay still as you squeeze and relax your ass cheeks.

Giddy-Up Cowgirl Part 2—The Reverse Cowgirl

This is a new spin on a favorite classic. You'll ride into the blissful sunset in this daring position—plus your lover will get an eyeful too!

Assume the Position:

Mount your lover facing away from him, so your back is to him. He can either be lying down on his back or propped up. Use your knees to thrust back against your partner for the ultimate penetration.

The Ample Advantages

- This position allows for deeper sensations and makes an orgasm even more likely than in a standard woman-on-top position since your lover's cock is at a better angle to hit your G-spot.
- While it provides your lover with an excellent view of your behind, as in the Doggy Style position, you are still in control of the thrusting and depth of penetration.
- Your lover can spank and grab your butt or wrap his arms around you, caress your breasts, and stimulate your clit, or you can do these things to yourself!
- The Reverse Cowgirl is a favorite of porn directors. This little piece of carnal knowledge is sure to boost your sex-esteem, knowing you are performing such an X-rated move!

Titillating Techniques

- Tell your lover to keep his legs firm and tensed so you have something to easily bounce off. This will give you the extra momentum needed for deeper thrusts.
- If your lover is lying down while you're riding him reverse-style, hold onto his feet and thrust backwards. Holding his feet will give you more leverage and make your thrusts more deep and delicious!
- To indulge in some kinky endeavors, ask your lover to spread your cheeks apart, spank them, or rub a gloved, lubed thumb around your anus.

> A cowgirl's favorite accessory? A riding crop! It can add an element of genuine kink to your next sexventure!

Satisfying Stance—Standing

Stand at attention in this delicious position! All the strength and energy you exert will be worth it when you're put to orgasmic ease.

Assume the Position:

Have your lover squat slightly as you lower your body onto him, either facing forward or with him behind. If facing forward, he can rest you up against a wall as you wrap your legs around him. With him behind, he can lean you forward as you rest your hands against a wall for some lovely leverage—we're already wet thinking about it!

The Ample Advantages

- This position screams "powerful, urgent lovemaking!"
- Either way you crave this position, your lover has access to your most delicious parts.
- It's a fun challenge to take on with your lover!

Titillating Techniques

- If your lover has taken you from behind in this position, try bending over and holding your ankles. Then stand up so you are up against his chest. The sensation of your riding up his cock will rev up his lust.
- If this position is too challenging at first, try getting on your knees to test the waters.
- Ask your lover to grab your hips, and begin grinding against him in circular movements. If you're face-to-face, you'll enjoy seeing your breasts bounce, and if you're taken from behind, he'll love watching your ass wiggle. Plus, the stimulation will send you soaring.

> This position is the perfect beginning to any tryst. If you get tired from all the pumping and thrusting, you can easily move down to the floor for some down-and-dirty sexcapades.

Boobie Fucking

Talk about loving your body! Seductively ask your partner to make love to you in this unorthodox fashion, and his head will spin so hard he'll be seeing double!

Assume the Position:

Have your lover hold your breasts together around his cock as he gently thrusts in and out of your super cleavage.

The Ample Advantages

- This is enjoyable for both parties involved, especially if you have very sensitive breasts.
- Your lover gets to experience the thrilling feeling of having his penis wrapped in the delicate flesh of your breasts.

- He can tease and tantalize your nipples with his cock, a new sensation for both of you.
- You both get a steamy visual!

Titillating Techniques

- Keep your head down to watch his penis peeking out between your breasts. For some extra kink, lick and suck the tip of his cock on every upward thrust.
- When he's about to cum, he can direct his ejaculation so that he creates a "pearl necklace" around your throat.

> Is your lover carnally creative? Here are some other unorthodox places on your body for him to fuck: armpits, between butt cheeks, and inner thighs.

CARNAL CHANGEUPS

Porn vixens know the importance of changing positions during sex—that's why you always see so many postures interlaced throughout a porn movie. While you may want to limit your scene changes, an erotic assortment of positions can always maximize your pleasure. Variety is the spice of lust, after all!

I Want You This Way … Now!

Here are some telltale signs it's time to change positions:

- You want to stall your lover's ejaculation for just a little bit longer so you can catch up.
- You want to get into a position where your lover can thrust hard so he can finally blast off.
- When you need to change the depth, variation, or sensation of your own genital stimulation to get closer to orgasm or delay your orgasm for heightened pleasure.

- When you're craving more intimacy than that particular position is giving you (or wanting less!).
- You're developing a leg cramp. Ouch!
- You're feeling like your current position is not going to move you over the edge.
- You or your lover just want a different view!

Anal Sex

Fulfill your own naughty wishes by performing one of *the* most infamous acts ever! Anal sex, the act of stimulating the anus and penetrating the anal canal, is probably the most versatile vintage sex option since penetration can be performed on a woman *or* a man!

> Do not rapidly change positions just to impress your lover with your knowledge of the Kama Sutra. It is not sexy and not very conducive to orgasms.

The skin of the human anus and the anal canal are densely packed with as many sensory receptors as clits and cocks. The tissue lining the anal canal is also delicately thin, causing it to be extremely sensitive. It's as though our butts have been naturally wired to discover this exquisite satisfaction!

While theorists, politicians, and religious groups may preach that anal sex is an unnatural form of intercourse, porn stars know the real truth. The anus wouldn't be such a pleasure-dome of mind-blowing orgasms if it wasn't meant to be penetrated. And men need to throw away their homophobic fears. Desiring anal sex does not make them gay. Desiring anal sex makes them sexually forward, and that's what all women want in their man!

Kiss My Ass—Rimming

As with any classic porn move, you should always start with a little smooching! Rimming is the act of kissing, licking, and nuzzling the outer edges of the anus, which

> Anal sex is *dirrrty*—not dirty. Your rectum is not a storage facility, so there should be little if any waste in your anal canal. However, if you would like added peace of mind, clean your anus with a soapy washcloth before sex (be sure to rinse well) and keep baby-wipes on hand during the act.

are packed full of nerve endings. There is method to this, especially for newbies, which should be strictly followed. Porn vixens suggest these steps:

- Do a rub/rub/rest, rub/rub/rest technique when first nuzzling your lover's anus with your finger or nose. This allows you to demonstrate how great anal play can feel without diving right in!
- Begin kissing and licking the area so that the nerve endings are not only stimulated but your lover can also feel your hot breath and wet lips in that area of their body.

> It is important that you use lots of lube when it's time for anal penetration because your anus is not self-lubricating like your vagina. Have fun flavored lubes available for this special event, like watermelon or chocolate. If this is your first time, get some cherry lube to be cheeky!

You can enjoy this erotic delight on its own, or you can use it as a great segue to actual anal penetration.

Perfect Penetration

Just as with any other great sex act, anal sex should include a cunnilingus or fellatio warm-up so your lover is thoroughly aroused even before you get to their back door. Here are some other essential steps to follow as penetration ensues. These apply to both men and women, so if you're on the receiving end, hand this to your lover to read.

- Make sure your lover is in a comfortable position, lying flat on the bed with her or his ass elevated on top of a pillow, or lying on one side.
- Begin by seductively pulling both ass cheeks apart and by doing so, gently stretching the skin in that area. This sensation is highly erotic, first because of the numerous nerve endings being stimulated and second because this is not an everyday, every-fuck, sensation.
- Rub your thumb over the anus in a similar fashion to when you were rimming. Kiss and lick this area. Use the tip of your tongue to delve into the tiny opening.
- Liberally apply lube to the area and to your finger. Push the tip of your thumb into your lover's anus to the first knuckle.
- If your lover's sphincter tightens, stop until it relaxes. Then proceed.
- Gradually upgrade. Use your thumb, then two fingers, then a medium-sized dildo, and then a penis or strap-on. This can take one trial or months of work. Don't get discouraged. The orgasms are worth the patience.
- Start penetration slowly (and men, use a condom!). Don't force it. Let the one who is receiving control the depth of penetration and speed of thrusting.

- If the woman is on the receiving end, porn vixens suggest clitoral stimulation during anal sex (either of you can do this). It can help keep the anal sensation from becoming too intense. It also connects anal and genital stimulation and heightens back-door satisfaction. Likewise, men will find that having their cock stroked greatly intensifies the pleasure.
- If your partner asks for more lube, give it to them! Pulling out to add lube actually intensifies the whole experience since the first inches of the rectum are where the strongest sensations lie, so multiple insertions feel grand!
- Remember, anal sex is more about penetration than friction. So, as always, keep adding that lube on for more wet and wild fun!

> Want a way to convince your man that anal sex is for him? Let him know that his prostate gland gets stimulated through anal sex, which can add significantly to his enjoyment and which ultimately leads to earth-shattering orgasms! Knowledge is sexual power!

Assume the Anal Position

Now that you've discovered the spectacular practice of anal sex, you'll need to find the best position for it. Our porn stars list their favorite positions to give and receive back-door pleasure:

- On hands and knees in the Doggy-Style stance
- Standing up while bent over

> Never double dip! Don't engage in anal sex and then begin vaginal sex without changing the condom. While your rectum is clean, there is a slight chance it contains a common bacterium called E. coli. The risk is not worth the pain that may ensue. Don't be a fool—wrap your tool, repeatedly if need be.

- Spooning
- Reverse Cowgirl, especially after a striptease!

HOT HOUSEHOLD POTENTIAL

While porn vixens have sex in the most exotic locations on earth, they know there's no place like home. Here are some of their steamy hot-spot suggestions for you, next time you're craving some domestic sex:

- Take a nice hot bath with your partner. Then make your own natural steam! Fill the bathtub halfway with warm water, mount your lover, and hold onto the sides for stability. Or have your lover enter you from behind, and use the showerhead to direct water onto your clit and his penis for additional stimulation.
- Sit on a loaded washer or dryer and have your lover enter you. Then hit "start" for some serious fireworks. The added rocking motion of these machines will help catapult you over the edge.
- Have your lover enter you from behind while standing in front of the window. Let your exhibitionism excite you!
- Do it Doggy Style on the couch while watching some fantastic porn—talk about an interactive movie!

See It to Believe It!
Favorite educational love making videos:
The Complete Guide to Sexual Positions—Sinclair Intimacy Institute, 1995, 60 minutes
Creative Positions for Lovers: Beyond the Bedroom— Ultimate, 2000, 60 minutes

The Guide to Advanced Sexual Positions—Sinclair Intimacy Institute, 1995, 27 minutes

Ordinary Couples, Extraordinary Sex Series—Sinclair Intimacy Institute, 1994, 60 minutes.

Sexual Ecstasy for Couples—Libido Films, 1997, 62 minutes

Nina Hartley's Guide to Anal Sex—Nina Hartley, 1995, 60 minutes.

Bonus Tip: Always remember: There is sexual freedom and awakening in the knowledge that you can perform X-rated moves to enhance your and your lover's carnal pleasure.

Forbidden Fruits

How to Indulge in the Tantalizing Taboo of Fetishes

Is sex dirty? Only if it's done right.

—Woody Allen

Even mainstream America seems to be jumping on the randy wagon as bondage, spanking, and S/M are becoming sexually acceptable in this new age of kink. Still, many women shy away from indulging in the fantastic world of fetishes, fearing they will be labeled as "one of those dirty girls."

Why let the dirty girls have all the fun? It's time to push the bedroom boundaries, accept your x-rated desires, and realize how sexually liberating it can be to be dirty! Embrace this new glorious sexual movement with open arms and open legs. Follow our next set of scandalous secrets, and you'll discover just how good it feels to be so bad!

One easy way to uncover which fetish works for you is through pornography itself. We can use porn films to introduce our lovers to any fetishes we desire to explore but have always been too shy to try. Just pop in the DVD, watch the scintillating scene on the screen, and then turn to your partner and say "Doesn't that look like fun?!"

If that is too sexually forward for you, you can also just browse for movies together at your local porn store. Take notes as you see which videos your lover picks up and investigates. You'll quickly discover what he's itching for!

In the meantime, here are a few starter fetishes to explore.

This Little Piggy Got It On

A foot fetish is one of the most popular of all sexual fetishes, tracing back centuries in history, even to Chinese foot binding.

Foot fetishes are still common today and are very much up-to-date. The indulgence incorporates your favorite sexual actions—kissing, licking, sucking, and caressing—so it's an easy addition to your sexual repertoire. It is also the most versatile of fetishes since it can be enjoyed as part of foreplay, postplay, and during-play. However you look at it, it's a world of pleasure for you and your lover!

> Before engaging in any foot fetish, remember to get a delicious pedicure. This way you'll be sure your toes are in tip-top shape, and instead of worrying about their appearance, you can sit back and relish the moment.

Head Over Heels

There are countless ways you can worship your lover's beautiful feet. You and your lover both can indulge your inner foot-freak with these naughty porn-star secrets:

- Massage your lover's foot, concentrating on the arch and each toe.
- Rub little circles on the inside of your lover's heel, just below the anklebone—not too light, or it will tickle too much. This will get their entire lower half tingling.

- Start kissing your lover's ankle, then kiss down the bridge of his foot, and finally kiss each individual toe.
- Lick your lover's toes, making sure you get the tip of your tongue between each delicious crevice.
- Suck his toes as though you were sucking a small hard candy.

Taking Care of Him

- Remember, your hands are not the only appendages that can help get his rocks off. Give him a foot job and jerk his way to bliss!

Taking Care of Her

- He can use his feet to worship you, too! Allow him to massage certain areas of your body, including your breasts, nipples, and pussy, with his feet only.

Fun Fetish

Whether you're on the giving or receiving end of this fantastic fetish, there's an assortment of items you can wear to experience new sensations. The skin at the bottom of your feet is very delicate and full of nerve endings. Therefore, various fabrics and materials will send different thrilling sensations down your spine. Wear some of these items next time you're craving some serious foot action.

- Stilettos
- Leather Boots
- Knee-High Socks
- Silk Stockings
- Toe Rings

BADASS BONDAGE

While you may think bondage in pornography is used to emphasize one lover's dominance over another, all the silk scarves, leather, and handcuffs actually allow you to be sexually generous. You get to display how ravenous you are for your lover's body and can tease and tantalize them without requiring reciprocation. While your partner is tied up, you get to prove that, at that moment, you're in this purely for their pleasure.

> There is a rumor out there that some women can orgasm from foot stimulation alone. Take time to discover if you're one of them!

There are a variety of provocative practices you can partake in after you've tied up your lover. Read the naughty suggestions from the sexperts themselves:

- Decide how badly your lover has misbehaved and calculate your level of reprimand. Is this a blindfolded or non-blindfolded offense?
- Tease your partner with light kisses and touches. Run feathers up and down her/his body.
- Fondle her/his nipples through a silk scarf.
- Vary the pattern of strokes and kisses, from deeply passionate to gentle caresses. Keep your lover guessing!
- Focus on pleasure points like nipples, inner thighs, ears, neck, and the line from the navel down to the genitals.
- While you're in control of the next move, play coy and seductive with your partner to heighten the anticipation.
- Gently scratch your nails up and down your lover's body.
- Intersperse lots of genital contact to keep things hot!
- If your lover is not blindfolded, masturbate in front of them. The visual stimulation will drive them crazy with lust!

- Bring your lover to the brink of orgasm, then pull back and begin the tantalizing teasing once more.
- Ladies, drag your nipples along his body; gents, use your cock and/or balls.
- Tantalize your lover with your tongue!
- Start having intercourse, and when it seems your lover is on the brink of orgasm, stop and begin kissing her/him gently to prolong the ultimate release.
- Finally, unleash an orgasm, either orally or through intercourse!

And what if you're the one tied up? There is a lot of pleasure in store for you! Not only are you admired and lavished with attention, there is a feeling of eroticism in the helplessness and anticipation associated with bondage.

> Next time you're craving a more brazen bondage technique, have your lover brush his cock and balls over your face. Demand that he press the bulb of his penis on your mouth and nose. This will be a very powerful rush for both of you.

Remember, being on top doesn't necessarily determine who is in charge. Next time you're tied up, call out orders for your lover to perform. Then sit back and fully enjoy sitting in the director's chair!

Bondage Don'ts

Bondage is something you should only practice with a partner you fully trust. Here are some other things to keep in mind before you get all tied up.

- Never allow anyone to restrain you by the neck. While it might be something that gets your juices flowing, it is too potentially dangerous. Opt for a pretty choker necklace or dog collar for the same sensation without the fear.

- Don't play rough or tough. Bondage is for the mutual enjoyment of lovers involved. (If you like it rough, see the next section on sadomasochism.)

- Never leave a bound person unattended, however briefly. As Murphy's Law would have it, whatever could go wrong at that time will go wrong.

EROTIC SPANKING

You've tied up your lover, teased him till he couldn't take it anymore, and then had your naughty way with him. It's time you were punished for all your wicked behavior!

The new age of kink has made erotic spanking not only sexually acceptable but actually expected at some point in one's lovemaking session. It takes playful sex to a new level, and makes both parties blissfully happy. Your lover gets to view the quiver of your flesh as he slaps your bottom, while you get to feel him caress a body part that may not usually get a lot of attention. You both get to experience some sizzling skin-to-skin contact.

The following are the scandalous steps to an erotic spanking session with a tantalizing twist:

- Keep your panties/boxers on, or bare it all!

> Take bondage to the next level. Next time a silk scarf or blindfolds are brought into the bedroom, try this kinky master/slave fantasy. Have your lover bring you to the brink of orgasm over and over again. Then have him masturbate and cum on your breasts or stomach. Order him to untie you and use the cum as lubricant to bring yourself to orgasm. Make sure he watches this visual treat!

- Remember to never hit too hard. That is the quickest way to kill the mood.
- First caress the flesh and then begin with quick, light slaps.
- Begin slapping with a firmer touch.
- Relax your wrist so your hand works like a paddle.
- Spread your fingers when you spank, instead of holding them together. It creates a totally different sensation.
- Remember that hitting the same spot over and over will produce a bruise and an upset lover—very counterproductive.
- Read the signs. A wiggly butt is satisfied with the splendor of spanking. Clenched cheeks are a sign that you may need to lighten up.
- Sometimes a sensual slap is just the thing. Other times a stronger measure is called for. Take your cues off the circumstances of the moment.
- *Never* spank in anger.

> If you want to experiment with more adventurous kink, spread his ass cheeks with one hand and then softly spank his anal area with two to three fingers of the other hand. Then ask for this fantastic fetish to be performed for you in return.

When Behaving Bad Feels So Good

Whether during foreplay or during the deed, you should always partake in the opportunity to spank your lover. The spontaneity of an invigorating spanking can be delightful in any position to which your randy romp takes you. However, the following tend to be the most pleasurable positions:

- Over the knees or across the lap
- Lying face-down on a bed
- Bent over the back of a chair

- Bending forward, hands on knees
- Kneeling on a bed or an ottoman, or on the floor on all fours

Paddle Pleasure

Tired of using your hands? Want to get carnally creative? Visit your local porn store for some fuzzy paddles or hardcore whips. However, if you're itching for some kinky sex on a whim, use these following everyday household items!

> Spanking can be taken outside the bedroom too! Playfully spank your lover while they are making dinner, holding the door open for you, or simply walking away from you. This flirty slap will help you both stay sexually connected during the day and build up the sexual anticipation for later that night.

- Paddles
- Rulers
- Hairbrushes
- Belts
- Kitchen Spatulas
- Canes
- Wooden Spoons
- Leather Gloves

> Remember to try out any item on yourself before you spank your lover with it, to ensure that it feels great!

Playful Punishment—Oh, Papi!

Use the following classic scenarios to heighten the erotic power behind your next scintillating spanking session:

- Naughty School-girl or-boy/Teacher
- Mommy/Daddy
- Master/Slave
- French Maid/Cheating Husband
- Tarzan and Jane

WHIPS AND LEATHER AND CHAINS ... OH MY!

Not all sadomasochism is about whips and leather—unless you want it to be! It can be as kinky or simply sensual as you desire. However, underneath it all, S/M is simply a power exchange between consensual lovers. The power games you decide to play depend on how sexually adventurous and/or experienced you are. If you are an enthusiastic novice ready to dive into this fantastic fetish, there are some warm-up drills you'll need to follow. Even if you're an S/M pioneer, it may be time to go back to the badass basics and relearn a thing or two.

> Agree to some ground rules with your lover before you engage in any sex games, such as not inflicting any deep pain, not leaving marks, setting a time limit to playing, and designating roles ahead of time. Make sure the basic boundaries are set so you know when you're pushing them further!

The Basics

Underneath the leather masks and metal-studded collars, S/M is about sexual dominance and submission, and there are randy benefits to be had from whichever role you choose. Read the following stimulating secrets to make the most of your performing role.

Steamy Surrender

Many women find it degrading to take a submissive position because of lessons learned from our grandmothers, mothers, and those women's studies classes we took in college. We've been told that women have submitted to men long enough, and that now is the time to rise above their dominance and reach equality.

Our porn stars are not suggesting you let equal rights fall by the wayside. In fact, they are not suggesting you submit to your lover at all. In the submissive role in S/M play, you are simply submitting to your own pleasure.

It takes a confident and independent individual to willingly surrender control of her own body. But the delight and satisfaction that is associated with giving someone else the reins to your arousal is not just a porn-star experience, it can be yours, too.

The Benefits

You get to wear some very cute and sexually appealing outfits! Porn stars list their top five favorite costume items for raunchy role-playing:

- Collars: These are the ultimate symbol of ownership. But remember, wearing a collar does not signify degradation; in fact it can confer a feeling of being cherished. You can purchase any collar at a pet store or specialty shop. More coy coquettes suggest a ribbon collar or a choker. Have your lover kiss your neck before putting it on you, to affirm the affection behind this sexual symbol.
- Stilettos: It is a simple fact that no one can run fast in spiked heels, so these sexy accessories reinforce an idea of temporary helplessness. Plus, they make your legs look amazing and make you feel hot as hell!
- Corsets: These laced-up numbers are restrictive, playing on the submissive role, and yet are flattering to your stomach and breasts. What better way to be tied up and under control?!
- Cuffs: Accessories like faux-fur lined wrist cuffs, hand-

cuffs, leather bracelets, and gold bangles all give the illusion that you are being held captive. The image alone can incite feelings of primal lust.

- Garter Belts: These sexy little items not only give off a restrictive vibe, keeping your panty hose up and your legs entrapped, they also allow for a delicious patch of skin to be exposed right where your pleasure zone starts!

The submissive role is not about just lying there looking pretty. Porn stars suggest speaking up next time you're playing the dutiful and acquiescent love slave ...

- Say things like, "I like to be held down when you fuck me," "I really love it when you pull my hair and make me go down on you," or "Please tell me how naughty I've been." Use your imagination.
- Ask permission before you do anything ... Can I put you in my mouth? Can I suck you long and hard? Can I make you cum?
- Play a sexual variation of Simon Says. If you forget to say "Sir" or "Madam" any time you speak or make a request, your lover gets to give you a little spanking!

If you're looking for more than a speaking role in your lovemaking game, here are some classic love-slave services you can provide for your partner ...

- Washing your lover's back in the tub
- Brushing his/her hair
- Shaving his/her genitals
- Helping him/her undress
- Perform oral services with no expectation of immediate reciprocation.

While you may originally have cringed at the idea of acting submissive during a spicy tryst, after reading these saucy secrets from the sexperts themselves, you can see there is much to gain from taking the passive role. Not only do you get to allow yourself to be super affectionate to your lover, you also cultivate your sexual skills and gain practice in the art of giving pleasure as an end in itself.

> The words "no" and "stop" are frequently used in S/M as part of a fantasy and often lose their real meaning. Before engaging in any S/M activities, always choose a *safe word* that you and your lover agree will be a signal to stop whatever you're doing. Think of a random word that would have nothing to do with your sex game, like "peanuts" or "pennies," and say it if you get uncomfortable and really do want to stop.

Sweet and Dandy Domination

It's time to take the reins and give him a rush—not just the rush of taking the initiative but of taking full control of the entire sexual romp. After you master these next porn star skills, he'll be begging for more.

The Benefits

Just as you dressed the part of the sultry submissive, you can also put on the costume of the delicious dominatrix. While dominatrices are often portrayed in latex and leather, there are items right in your everyday wardrobe that are just as effective for dirty dressing:

- Lingerie and heels
- Well-fitted work suit and glasses
- Corset, short skirt, and knee-high boots

While you had some limited permission to talk as a submissive, as the dominant player you have the starring role. You control the actions, the pace, and all the fucking. It is important to keep your orders short and simple, to highlight the aloof and controlling character you are portraying. But don't go overboard and just start barking orders at your partner. Sex games are supposed to be enjoyable, not humiliating.

Porn stars suggest giving these carnal commands as your submissive lover is assuming the position:

- "Give me your other end."
- "Take off your clothes."
- "Get on top."
- "Crawl over there."
- "Open your legs."
- "Fuck me now!"

Or, if you're a gentler leader:

- "You're being very pleasurable tonight. Keep up the good work."
- "You look beautiful on your knees."
- "You may take me now."
- "See how excited you get me?"

> It is very important not to get lost in the dominant role. You are his/her lover first and a dominatrix second. With the possible exception of real hardcore masochists, no one wants to be dominated by a bitch.

While the dominant player does a lot of commanding, they also get to do a lot of touching, kissing, sucking, and fucking. Follow these next steps to see just how good it can be when you get to do all the work.

- Take the initiative and undress your lover as quickly or slowly as you'd like.

- Keeping in character as you tantalize and tease your lover, make sure your touch is firm, but not rough.
- Take pride in what you're doing. Make your lover say "thank you" after you perform even the tiniest tasks: "Thank you for nibbling my ear," "Thank you for sucking my penis," etc.
- Masturbate in front of your lover as if you were alone.
- You can either take the active role as the dominant player and fuck the submissive, or you can order the submissive to fuck you.

> Most S/M porn movies do not feature traditional fucking and climaxing. Make sure to correct this omission in your own personal experiments with this kinky technique. What better way to indulge in a new fetish then to have a happy ending.

For Advanced Lovers

There are numerous levels of S/M, and the riskier variations definitely can ignite some serious sexual fireworks. Beyond the basics lies sex that is a little more crazy and kinky, though not any less sensual.

Favorite XXX-Rated S/M scenarios:

- Tie up your lover and drip hot wax on key areas of her/his body.
- Wear a strap-on dildo and fuck your lover until he begs you to stop.
- Wear your highest knee-high boots and demand that he kiss and lick them.

> Many women crave randier and rougher sex just before their menstrual cycle. This is a great time to smolder the sheets with some experimental S/M.

- Sit in the Reverse Cowgirl position as you make love, and have your partner whip you to keep the momentum rocking.

See It to Believe It!

Some educational porn videos on S/M and other favorite fetishes:

Fetish FAQ Series—Bizarre Video, 2000, each film approximately 60 minutes

Learning the Ropes Series—Gen XXX, 1992, each film approximately 80 minutes

The Pain Game—Sunshine, 2000, 54 minutes

Tie Me Up—Academy of SM Arts, 2002, 52 minutes

Whipsmart—Good Vibrations/Sexpositive Productions, 2001, 82 minutes

The Fist, the Whole Fist, and Nothing but the Fist—Patrick Collins, 2000, 78 minutes

Nina Hartley's Guide to Swinging—Adam and Eve Productions, 1996, 73 minutes

Bonus Tip: Always remember: Do not judge before you indulge. You do not know that you won't enjoy something until you surrender to it fully.

Cumming Home

 HOW TO GET A HAPPY ENDING

Electric flesh-arrows traversing ... the body.
A rainbow of color strikes the eyelids. ... It
is the gong of the orgasm.

—Anaïs Nin

Laughter and orgasm are great bedfellows.

—John Callahan

It's the grand finale, the sweet release, the money shot, the
stuff movie magic is made of. How do you bring the glitz
and glamour of a porn orgasm into your bedroom?
Simple. You lay down some ground rules and practice,
practice, practice, until you get it oh-so right!

Orgasms are as unique and different as snowflakes and vary
in intensity. Some are large, powerful, and toe-curling.
Others (at least for women) are gentle and subtle, providing
a slight shiver of satisfaction. All are naturally beautiful.

However, porn stars know orgasms like the captain of a ship
knows the ocean. They are familiar with every wave, every
undulation, and every ripple an orgasm can generate. And
they know the secrets to riding those killer waves every single
time, one right after the other.

FOOLISHLY FAKING

The word "orgasm" comes from the Greek word *orgasmos*, which means "to swell" or "to be excited." However, there is nothing swell or exciting about faking an orgasm. It is patronizing to your lover and unhealthy for the state of your well-being. Besides, lying is not an intimate act. Your lover will never learn how to give you what you really need, and you'll end up lying passively by as each possible body-quaking orgasm is lost. Stand up for what is rightfully yours, take your lover by the hand, and lead him into the bedroom.

ORGASM ESSENTIALS

Now that faking has been officially abolished from your sexual vocabulary, you'll need to learn which elements are essential for guaranteeing that you hit the high note time and time again. You are in luck—here are the three secret keys to orgasmic satisfaction.

G-Spot Stimulation: The G-spot is a tiny spongy area of nerve tissue located about halfway between the back of the pubic bone and the top of a woman's cervix. Have your lover try to locate it by inserting a finger into your vagina and making a "come hither" movement. Direct stimulation of this area produces blissful results that feel like an internal shudder.

Clitoral Stimulation: Your clitoris is a tiny bulb of flesh between your vaginal lips that is full of nerve endings (about 8,000, as opposed to the roughly 4,000 in a cock). This area is usually stimulated through manual or oral measures but can be put in play during sex as well. A clitoral orgasm can generate electric sensations throughout your lower region.

Emotional Stimulation: There is no doubt that having a deep emotional connection to your lover is essential to achieving the deepest of orgasms. Orgasms are basically an unleashing of control of your body. You must have that emotional attachment and trust with your partner in order to truly let go and indulge in your most earth-shattering orgasms.

Sure-Fire Blastoffs

Not all positions incorporate the three keys to satisfaction we've just covered—especially not the Kama Sutra, bend-like-a-pretzel ones. Thank goodness for blissful basics. Here are our silver-screen vixens' five favorite sex positions that include at least two of the three orgasm essentials, to ensure mind-blowing, bed-rattling orgasms time and again.

Downward Dog

This is an orgasmic twist on a classic yoga position. Instead of balancing yourself on all fours, lie on your stomach, lift your butt slightly, and have your lover enter you from behind. He can prop himself up as if doing push-ups, or lie directly on top of you as he thrusts. The depth of penetration allows for an increased amount of friction and direct stimulation to your G-spot. You can also rub your clit against the bed sheets for added stimulation. Either way you'll end up with one out-of-this-world orgasm.

Tantalizing Table Top

Craving an orgasm with your next meal? Lie on your back on the dinner table with your butt near the edge. Have your lover enter you while standing between your legs. Raise one leg over his shoulder. This will not only allow for deeper penetration and direct stimulation of your G-spot, it also will give him a beautiful view of all your curves. Plus, his hands will be free to stroke your breasts, inner thighs, and clit. To increase your odds of having an orgasm in this position, clench and lift your butt. This will add to the pelvic tension and blood flow to the area.

Ride Him Cowgirl

Usually women are guaranteed an orgasm when astride their lovers. However, by adding a 180-degree twist to your next on-top adventure, you can increase your odds of achieving satisfaction. While on top, swing around into the Reverse Cowgirl position so you are looking at your partner's feet. Hold your legs together, feet flat between his legs. This will not only make the fit even tighter and give way to deeper sensations, it also allows for increased G-spot stimulation. Also, in this position you can pleasure your own clit as your partner thrusts upward and strokes your body. All these elements can come together to create a very explosive orgasm.

The Spoon

Use the spoon position to reach a blissful orgasm. You both simply lie on your sides, with you in front of your lover. Have him enter you from behind. Instead of enjoying his usual in-and-out thrusting, however, ask him to stay inside of you and gently move back and forth against the insides of your vagina.

This will provide constant simulation to your G-spot, and the position allows for the emotional connection also needed to achieve a great orgasm.

Liberating Lap Dance

Unleash your wildest orgasms with this next position. With your lover sitting in a chair or propped up in bed, straddle him so that you are face-to-face. Instead of moving up and down, though, sway back and forth so you're rubbing your clit against him. There are many pleasures to be found in this position: your breasts will be wonderfully aligned with his mouth; if you lean back a bit, he can play with your clit and you'll get deeper G-spot stimulation; and you can kiss passionately to stay emotionally connected. All these benefits can only lead to a liberating orgasm.

During sex, as your lover climaxes, tug his hair lightly. This will flood him with endorphins, which will electrify his orgasm.

Tips, Tricks, and Titillating Techniques

Here are some other industry secrets to ensure you'll have orgasms in some of your other favorite sex positions.

- Clamp down on his penis with your vaginal muscles. When you bear down, you'll experience deeper sensations.
- When lying down during sex, push your feet against a wall. This tightens your body and can help you move around to enhance sexual pleasure.
- Lie flat on your back with your legs together, hips flexed up, and your guy straddling you. This tightens your love muscles, so you'll have an easier time achieving orgasm.

- Quick panting at the beginning of an orgasm rushes oxygen to your brain and intensifies the pleasure.
- You or your lover can pinch your nipples as you cum. The sensation will intensify your orgasm.
- If you think you aren't getting enough sensation during intercourse, ease up on the lubrication.
- Gently pulling your lover's testicles away from his body can lengthen his orgasm.
- Have your lover move in slow motion when he's about to blast off. It will cause his orgasms to be more powerful.
- Drinking two glasses of wine can loosen any inhibitions you may have about stripping down and letting your vixen out. Limit your alcoholic intake, however, since too much booze can desensitize your body to your lover's touch.
- Health specialists believe that ginseng can heighten your orgasmic experience.

Carnal Conditioning

Another trade secret to never faking an orgasm again is knowing exactly what *your own* right moves are. What better way to learn what gets you over the edge than doing in-depth studies and conducting extensive experimental solo sessions? Figure out what works for you by caressing your breasts, thighs, and everything in between when you have an afternoon (or even a few minutes) alone. As Jenna Jameson recommends: "Masturbate daily. It [not only] releases energy, exercises your love muscles, and helps you master your vagina, [but also] you'll learn what your body needs and [you'll] never have to fake it."

Experiment with the following:

- Different textures can be a tantalizing turn-on. Find out which ones work for you. Use silk scarves, a terry washcloth, or one of his cotton tee shirts to rub against your clitoris, inner thighs, and breasts.
- Experiment with your vibrator. Use it while in different positions. Find out which ones give you the quickest orgasms, or the most powerful ones, and discover the positions that turn you on but don't put you over the edge. If your carnal urges are strong and you don't desire a sensitive touch, pull back the hood of your clitoris and put the vibrator right on your sweet spot. If you're super sensitive, keep your panties on.
- If you want to clean up your dirty act, get your butt in the shower. More specifically, get under the faucet, run the water directly on your pussy, and test various water intensities to see which one brings you to orgasm.
- Study your vagina. Having an intimate understanding of your most private area will help you appreciate both its beauty and function as a sex organ. Then take that empowering knowledge into the bedroom.

> It has been documented that a small percentage of women can reach orgasm through nipple stimulation alone and that some men can orgasm with only testicle stimulation. Have some fun investigating if you or your lover are one of the lucky few.

EARTH-MOVING ORGASMS

Now that you know the basics for guaranteeing orgasms, here are some advanced techniques to guarantee ground-shattering fun.

The Sexy Twist to the Missionary Position

While the missionary position is often for beginners or those of us who are shy about making love, there are still explosive orgasms to be found in this rudimentary position.

- When you sense that he is near orgasm, grab a hold of his hipbones or butt and rock him back and forth or side to side. By controlling the direction of his pelvis movements you can also control the depth and speed of his thrusting. Also, it will give him a powerful feeling that you are pulling the orgasm out of him.

Butterfly Kisses

Women generally prefer lighter touching to get them aroused. But what about using lighter touches to get you off, too? The following technique will have you moaning for more butterfly kisses. Have your lover follow these instructions:

- Caress your lover's genitals orally and manually until she is near orgasm. Shift gears and then use your hands and mouth to gently kiss and caress other areas of her body such as her breasts and inner thighs. Then go back to genital caresses. When she is again near orgasm, move your mouth to other parts of her body. Alternate between direct genital and nongenital stimulation until she is so aroused that you can bring her to orgasm by just sucking one nipple and gently stroking her inner thigh. She will experience a whole-body orgasm that is out of this world.

The Grand Finale

Men often are considered lucky because an orgasm is nearly always inevitable at the end of sex play. However, their orgasms may vary in depth as well. To make your lover blast off like never before, follow this secret to a full-body orgasm.

• Orally stimulate your lover's penis almost to the point of orgasm. Stop suddenly, and then shift your attention to his balls, inner thighs, or other parts of his body. Repeat. Do this until you notice he seems almost in pain. Then hold his thighs apart and lower your mouth to his perineum (the area between his anus and the base of his scrotum). Flick your tongue rapidly across this area and then insert a finger or thumb into his anus as you continue to flick your tongue. This type of stimulation will bring him an orgasm that sends explosive vibrations throughout his entire body.

> Some women have the ability to think themselves to orgasm. Quick, get some naughty thoughts running through your mind and find out if you're one of them!

The Myth of the Simultaneous Orgasm

Remember that having orgasms together is a rarity, and not having them together doesn't mean you and your partner lack sexual compatibility, emotional connection, or love. Simultaneous orgasms are most often a silver-screen special effect, just like aliens or hobbits.

That doesn't mean it will never happen. Just treasure it when it does, but never ever dismiss your unsynchronized orgasms. An orgasm on your own can be just as powerful as one simultaneous with your lover. Be selfish for those few minutes and ride alone on the waves to bliss. The sight and sounds of your unbridled passion will drive your lover crazy.

That said, there are a few secret tips on how to promote simultaneous orgasms. Follow these steps and see if you can create some of that movie magic for yourself.

- Many women need direct clitoral stimulation to orgasm, and often intercourse doesn't provide that touch. Therefore your O-face may only come out during manual or oral sex. In order to reach orgasm together while fucking, have your lover use extra lube, to imitate the wetness of his mouth. Have him enter only halfway in the beginning, simulating the shallow penetration of tongue and fingers. Or saddle up and get on top. This position allows the most clitoral stimulation, and you can move your pelvis in circles to intensify the sensations.
- Since men tend to reach climax before women, let him know you need a head start. Ask him for an extended amount of foreplay and then have him tease you orally for at least ten minutes. Just as you feel you are nearing the edge of bliss, have him enter you. This way, you are already fully aroused and need only some penetration to get your rocks off, and you can co-climax with perfect timing.
- When you're on top and you can sense that your lover is close to orgasm, stop your movements for a few minutes. A small cooling-off period can enable you both to reach simultaneous climax together once you start bucking up again.
- Always keep a vibrator on hand. You can use it when you need a little added stimulation to get you and your lover

over the edge. Just place it on your clit and the vibrations may make you both explode simultaneously.

- Some people believe that simultaneous orgasms occur only when a couple is in harmony. However, we don't suggest relying on the hocus-pocus of trying to read each other's minds. Instead, we suggest talking with your partner and letting him know your orgasm readiness with a simple "hold on a second" or "slow down, I'm not there yet." This way you can hold off orgasm until you are ready to cum together. We would never want to stifle your creative ability, so if you want to come up with seductive ways to communicate this information during sex that fan the flames of your sex play, all the better!

> Most men are not just in it for themselves. A major part of their overall sexual satisfaction is the ego boost they get from being able to make their partners climax.

MULTIPLE ORGASMS

Only one-third of women have multiple orgasms, and an even smaller percentage have them on a regular basis. The good news is that all women are capable of having multiple orgasms and luckily there are great tricks you can learn to condition your body to produce these marvelous explosions. All it takes is a little bit of practice, a lot of loving, and the willingness to orgasm over and over and over again.

Are You My Type?

Before you can refine your skills and become a multiorgasmic woman, you need to learn the types of multiple orgasms there are. Each type listed below can be reached through intercourse, oral sex, or manual stimulation (or with a little bit of all three!).

Compounded singles: Each orgasm is distinctly separated by some amount of time. For example, you achieved one orgasm and have cooled down and then achieved another one.

Sequential multiples: These types of orgasms are very close together, from one to ten minutes apart. There is little interruption in sexual arousal. For example, you achieve one orgasm while your lover is orally stimulating you and then achieve another during intercourse.

Serial multiples: The orgasms are separated only by seconds or minutes, with no interruption in stimulation.

Blended multiples: This is a mix of two or three orgasms of differing lengths and intensities. It is normal for a woman who is multiorgasmic to experience different types of orgasms during one randy romp session.

Get Yourself Going

A woman doesn't become multiorgasmic overnight—she does have to put some effort into it. Here are some tried-and-true conditioning techniques that will help develop your ability to cum over and over again.

- Women who are not comfortable touching themselves are less capable of having multiple orgasms. Stroke yourself during intercourse, or take his hand and show him how you want to be stroked. After your first orgasm, don't stop the stimulation. You'll feel another orgasm building up behind the first one.

- Some women need to have both clitoral stimulation and vaginal stimulation in the G-spot region to experience multiple orgasms. Discover if you're one of them by having your lover stimulate the front wall of your vagina with his fingers while he's eating you out. Or, you or your lover can stimulate your clitoris during intercourse.

> A hint that it will be a multiorgasmic night: your first orgasm doesn't feel like a complete release. Chances are, you are so aroused that one orgasm isn't enough to release all your pent-up sexual tension. When this happens, hold on— it's going to be a bumpy ride!

THE KEGEL EXERCISE

Now that you know how to be multiorgasmic and have learned a few techniques to make your orgasms reach stellar heights, it's time to become acquainted with an exercise that keeps 'em coming.

Everyone is understandably concerned about physical health. Looking at the number of gyms popping up across the nation, the quantity of diet foods lining grocery store shelves, and the increased participation in yoga and exercise classes, health awareness is clearly sweeping the country. However, if you are concerned with the health of your orgasms, the only exercises worth their weight in sweat are called "kegels."

No Gym Membership Required

Kegel exercises develop the pubococcygeus (PC) muscles, which form part of the pelvic floor. Just tighten them (as if you need to go pee but have to hold it in) and then release. You can do Kegels anywhere; stuck in traffic, at the office, at a ball game, and even during foreplay. You can hold the muscles for as little or as long as you like before releasing. The exercises tighten your vagina while boosting blood flow to the area, which creates a warm and invigorating sensation. They also make a huge difference in your sexual performance and enjoyment. Whip your vagina into shape, and you'll be better able to quench your sexual appetite.

The Kegel Orgasm

Kegels aren't only for helping prepare for better sex. You can also do them *during* sex, to enhance the experience.

- Simply flex your PC muscles as he thrusts into you, and release as he pulls out. As you hold and release these muscles in time with his thrusting, you are also intensifying the sensations for your lover. As he gets closer to climax, you can begin to tighten and release these muscles in more rapid succession. As he orgasms, it will feel as if you are pulling the cum from his body into yours—a truly intense orgasmic experience for both of you.

> What to do when your lover cums before you have achieved orgasmic bliss? Have him either perform cunnilingus or manually stimulate you, or, if you are of a more kinky nature, have your lover kiss, stroke, and lick you as you masturbate yourself to orgasm.

Orgasm Interrupted

Once in a while your lover may lose his erection. *Do not* take the blame for this or blame him. Many things can cause a flaccid penis, such as consuming too much alcohol, excessive stress from work, or even performance anxiety. However, if you have a few tricks up your sleeve, male impotence can be a momentary problem.

Standing Ovation

In this move, take his cock firmly in your hand. Then place it in your mouth, moving the top third of his shaft in and out. Use your other hand to stroke his perineum with a "come hither" movement. As he becomes erect, swirl your tongue around his corona. You can also alternate between flicks, licks, and swirls, to add variety to the revival. Be sure to not take his penis too far into your mouth. By concentrating on his tip and the top third of his cock, you'll be able to pull off the suction needed to get him hard. He'll be sure to be giving you a standing ovation for your performance soon enough.

Giddy-Up

If he's able to get slightly erect but not hard enough for penetration, try this trick. Grasp the base of his penis firmly in one hand and use the head to stroke your own pussy. After a few minutes, lower your body onto his penis without letting go of your grip. With your PC muscles, grasp the first third of his penis, and contract your muscles to simulate the act of thrusting. If he remains soft, work in his entire

Do not get discouraged if your lovemaking doesn't always end with the big O. If you don't have an orgasm for two to three lovemaking sessions, the anticipated release will be that much more powerful and profound when you finally reach the point of no return. You will not only desire sex more strongly, but your orgasm will also be deeper than your normal, everyday orgasms.

penis, all the while using your PC muscles to bring yourself to orgasm. By the time he feels the internal spasms of your orgasm on his cock, he should be hard and ready to go for round two.

See It to Believe It!

Watch the following educational videos to see exactly how to achieve out-of-this-world orgasms:

Incredible G-Spot—Park Avenue Publishers, 1995, 60 minutes

Becoming Orgasmic—Sinclair Intimacy Institute, 1993, 83 minutes

Celebrating Orgasms—Pacific Media Entertainment, 1996, 60 minutes

The Guide to G-Spots and Multiple Orgasms—Sinclair Intimacy Institute, 1999, 60 minutes

Bonus Tip: Always remember: If you focus only on reaching the finish line, you won't have time to enjoy the thrill of the race.

Titillating and Tantalizing Toys

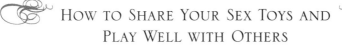 How to Share Your Sex Toys and Play Well with Others

> The best sex I have ever had was with my vibrator.
>
> —Eva Longoria

As a carefree child, you loved playing with toys, especially bright and shiny ones with all the bells and whistles. Why should that change now that you're a pleasure-seeking adult?!

Bringing sex toys into your sex-play shows your lover your mischievous side, not to mention your spicy, try-anything attitude. Plus, sex toys have the power to intensify your sexual enjoyment and promote positive erotic pleasure for you and your lover.

Our porn stars give you a sneak peek into their toy chests and tell you how to play nice while reaping bad-girl benefits.

Opening the Sex Toy Box

Too often, even sexually forward women shy away from introducing sex toys into their relationships because they don't want their partners to assume they are not sexually satisfied. However, porn stars understand the provocative power of sex toys. They know that bringing them into the bedroom does not express anything negative about the carnal abilities of you or your lover. On the contrary, sex toys can add new sensations to your sexual repertoire, enhance your sex life, and connect you more closely to your lover as you explore and experiment with new ways to share and enjoy pleasure.

Here are a few things to consider discussing before bringing in sex toys to play with under your own sheets:

- Let your lover know that your desire to use toys does not mean he is not an excellent lover. You each have individual wiring, and even Casanova might not be able to get you to hit that sweet high note. He actually can become an even more proficient lover by acquiescing to your vibrating desires.

- Sex toys are not for your pleasure alone. Assuage any toy-jealousy that may arise by educating him about the ways vibrators and dildos can also heighten his enjoyment (further details follow). Also, emphasize that you can't do this alone—to get your rocks off, you need him just as much as your toys.

- Reassure him that playing with sex toys does not make him gay or emasculate him, if that is what he

> You do not have to behave like a porn star to enjoy sex toys. Do not be insulted if your lover brings home a tantalizing toy, and don't assume you automatically have to shove it deeply into any orifice available to show your appreciation. Sex toys can be used subtly during sex play. And remember, he just wants to ensure you are experiencing the most pleasure possible. What could be sweeter than that?!

fears. Sex toys create erotic vibrations and motions, and the desire to experience these sensations is neither gay nor straight but is innately human.

VIBRATING TO BLISS

Vibrators can offer a world full of blissful orgasms. They not only help women discover what they need to blast off, they also help condition our bodies for multiple or simultaneous orgasms. Plus, with their diverse shapes, sizes, colors, and functions, they are fun items to bring into the bedroom when you are in an experimental mood. They offer a win-win solution to any relationship-rut problems!

Here is our porn-star list of the seven wonders of the vibrant vibrating world:

The Rabbit

This vibrator became famous overnight after a cameo in *Sex in the City*. Boy did Samantha know what she was talking about! This vibrator stimulates all the right spots, all at once. Insert the shaft into your vagina and press "play." The device will twirl and stimulate your G-spot, while the pearls at the base of the shaft stimulate the lower vagina. That cute little rabbit attached to the shaft packs a huge punch, too, stimulating your clit with its ears.

Randy Recommendation: Choose this vibrator when you're feeling experimental and want to achieve intense orgasms. In other words, this can be your everyday go-to vibrator!

The Pocket Rocket

This is the most discreet of vibrators, looking more like a lipstick tube than a provocative plaything. Apply it directly to your vulva and your clit for some strategic sensual stimulation. You'll be amazed at the amount of zing this teeny-tiny item can generate.

Randy Recommendation: Being travel sized, this vibrator is great for the on-the-go woman, and also is great for stimulating your lover's cock (read on to find out how!).

Hitachi Magic Wand

This vibrator is great for massaging your lower back and shoulders—and some other delicious areas. However, it is more powerful than other vibrators mentioned here and can take some time getting used to. It has two speeds and a robust internal motor. If you find it too powerful, fold a washcloth in half and place it over your pubic bone before applying. The real secret to this toy's pleasure is keeping it in slow motion. Move this vibrator across your vulva more slowly than you would normally deem necessary. You want to ensure that every nerve is blasting off, and if you move too quickly, you may not get that effect.

Randy Recommendation: Use it when you want instant, intense orgasms!

Talking-Head Vibrator

Need some extra-dirty talk when getting down and dirty? This vibrator is your ticket! Made of stunning blue or pink silicone, it has the same pearls at the end of the shaft and ears for clit stimulation that The Rabbit has, and it also has a voice-recorder computer chip that produces CD-quality sound. Record your own (or your lover's) dirty talk, or choose among prerecorded "fantasy chips"—French, Italian, or German lovers, or kinky dominatrix scenarios.

Randy Recommendation: It stimulates you, mind, body, and soul.

The Strap-On Vibrator

Ever wanted to enjoy the sensations of a vibrator but still have both hands readily available to wander elsewhere? Well, want no more. The Strap-On Vibrator is a small vibrator that is held in place against your clit with pretty, perfect straps. While it is not as powerful as other vibrators, it is also not as intrusive a toy. Since it's on the smaller side, you can easily introduce it next time you're making love, and he can enjoy the mild vibrations as well.

Randy Recommendation: Perfect for both parties in play!

The Natural Contours Vibrator

Designed by porn-star-turned-porn-director Candida Royalle, this vibrator fits the natural curve of your vulva and sends gentle vibrations throughout your vagina. Also, it is not created in man's phallic image but instead is shaped to satisfy your womanly needs.

Randy Recommendation: With its unobtrusive size and shape, this vibrator is perfect for a woman just beginning to experiment with sex toys.

Read more about Candida Royalle's directing experience in the Ultimate Visual Stimulation chapter later in this book. You'll soon understand why she's every woman's hero!

Eroscillator™

A revolutionary toy, this device doesn't vibrate but rather oscillates back and forth almost thirty-six hundred times a minute. Made with silicone and equipped with interchangeable heads, this is great for producing spine-tingling orgasms.

Randy Recommendation: Thirty-six hundred times a minute! Need we say more?!

> Always remember to clean all your toys after each use. This protects you from germs and bacteria, and keeps your toys shiny, sparkly, and in tip-top condition.

The "Play" Button

Though the use of vibrators may seem self-explanatory, here's how to get the most pleasure out of your toys. Follow these steps to orgasmic toy bliss:

- Press the vibrator against your clit. You can do this with silk panties on for gentler sensations, or if you're putting on a show for your lover!
- Experiment with varying pressures and speeds, and move the vibrator over your vulva, labia, clitoris, and surrounding areas, such as your inner thighs.
- Play with prolonging your orgasm. Once you feel you are on the brink, pull the vibrator away. This helps condition your body for stronger orgasms and can also

> If your lover wants to play with your toys, let him! Start your vibrator on a slow speed and run it along the shaft of his penis. As the hairs on his neck rise, press it against the base of his cock, his scrotum, and his perineum. If he's up for it, experiment with higher speeds and different pressures.

condition it for multiple orgasms, as discussed in the previous chapter.

Couple Vibrator Play

Vibrators are not just for you! Take the sharing skills you learned in grade school and bring them into the bedroom. Porn vixens suggest lovers use vibrators to tease each other unmercifully as a form of scintillating seduction and fore-play. Read their tips and tricks on how to vibrate together.

- Take turns giving each other sensual massages with your vibrator. Use it on the back, shoulders, legs, and everything in between. Move it up and down each other's bodies, and move it toward and away from each other's genitals.
- Or use it as an element of foreplay. Place the vibrator on your lover's cock to vary stimulation between oral and hand play.
- Stimulate your lover's perineum with a small vibrator during oral or manual lovemaking.
- Ask your lover to use the G-spot vibrator to stimulate you while in the 69 position.
- Use an anal vibrator while performing fellatio on your lover, or ask him to use one while eating you out. Use lots of lube for this, and remember to start slow. This play gives you the sensation of having a threesome without the negative emotional repercussions.
- Insert a wand-shaped vibrator between your bodies during inter-course. Your partner will feel

> Just as with anal sex, there is no double dipping with anal toy play. If you use a vibrator to stimulate your lover's anus, do not then use it on your vulva. For sanitary reasons, clean it or use another toy.

indirect vibrations throughout his penis while he is inside you, and you'll get some additional clit stimulation. These distinctly different sensations will send you soaring!

DECADENT DILDOS

Craving a toy that gives you the power to control the speed of thrusting and depth of penetration, rather than just having a vibrator vibrate you? We have the toy for you!

Dildos usually have the same phallic shapes as many vibrators but have no vibrating component. Many women prefer dildos to vibrators because they feel more like the real deal, since they are made from lifelike materials like silicone and are the actual sizes of real cocks. Consequently, playing with one actually feels like having real sex. Plus, they come in all shapes, colors, and styles, so you can have fun shopping to find the one that is perfect for you!

Porn stars suggest using dildos to not only stroke your vulva, labia, and clit as you would with a vibrator, but also for deeper penetration to achieve G-spot stimulation. Let your passion be your guide. You can go as gentle, rough, shallow, or deep as you like when indulging yourself with this titillating toy.

> Make sure you use a water-based lube when using a silicone dildo; silicone-based lubes will ruin the surface of the toy. Also remember not to bite into one in the heat of passion. The tiniest tear in silicone can result in a good clean break. Then the fun would be over for everyone!

Strap-On Dildos

While your lover has a phallic-shaped toy already attached to his delicious body, there are ways a strap-on dildo and a little bit of creativity can maximize your carnal chemistry! Remember, it pays to play well with others!

Put a little spin on your normal sexual roles, and have a naughty "what-was-that?!" experience.

Playing with strap-on dildos is perfect for the man who loves anal penetration. He gets to experience the thrill of anal stimulation while you get to take full control of the thrusting and experience a rush of power and lust. Plus, a dildo will definitely stimulate his prostate.

Having a strap-on attached also frees up your hands for other provocative pursuits, like reaching around and playing with his cock as you thrust into his back door.

Hair-Raising Harnesses

Go strap-on dildo shopping together at a local sex shop or online so you can decide which version of this sex toy will give both your libidos a real boost. Plus, viewing and/or reading about these toys can rev up your engines for some post-shopping nooky! Here are some booty-full basics about the equipment you'll need.

> As always with anal play, remember to use lots of water-based lube, and allow him to direct the depth and speed of penetration. Ask him to give you some erotic instructions to heat up the dirty talk, then take him with raw and animalistic passion.

- **Basic Harness:** This has adjustable straps that go around your waist and thighs with a spot to insert a dildo. Its simplicity makes it simply sexy!
- **G-String Harness:** With a lovely leather thong attached to a slim waistband and a single strap running up the center of your butt and over your clit, this strap-on will give your

lover a large hard-on and give you great stimulation at the same time!

- **The Jock Strap:** This dildo is attached to a waistband that has two straps passing around each thigh. It leaves your vagina exposed so your lover can reach his hands around his back to pleasure you as you give it to him right!

- **Vibrating Harness:** Oh my! This harness has two little vibrating pads attached, one next to your clit and one where the dildo comes out of the harness, for extra anal stimulation. It offers intense his-and-hers happiness!

> When surprising your lover with a sex toy, be sure not to just thrust it into any orifice available without some prior carnal communication. Some surprises are best discussed beforehand!

TOYS FOR THE BOYS

Just as there are sex toys geared specifically toward women, there are also toys made especially for our male lovers. Just as we may bring our favorite playthings into the bedroom to creatively spice up the moment, he should bring his toys too. Remember, sharing is carnally caring!

Jack-of-All-Trades

One of the most innovative toys of the sexual revolution is the Jack-off Sleeve. It is made either of cyber skin or super-stretchy silicone, and is formed in a flexible tube shape. The sleeve goes over your lover's penis and has a very soft and smooth texture, which is excitingly different than the feeling of hands. He can run it up and down his cock during a solo session, or he can ask you to manipulate it during foreplay.

Cock-A-Doodle-Do

Cock Rings are one of the most infamous of male sex toys. Made of rubber, silicone, leather, or metal, they fit snugly around a man's cock and balls. When he's hard, the cock ring prolongs his erection by constricting blood flow to this area and keeping blood in the penis shaft. This means he'll last longer under the sheets so you're able to blast off several times before he's ready to cum. Not only will you be fully sexually satisfied, he'll feel like a regular sex god!

> As noted, some cock rings are metal. However, beginners should go with rubber or adjustable versions with snaps or velcro, so if something goes wrong they are easily cut off or removed. Don't risk an embarrassing trip to the emergency room!

Feel the Vibrations

Add a little zing to your cock ring! A vibrating cock ring is normally a simple silicone ring attached to a vibrating torpedo and battery pack. There are two ways to play with this toy: stretch the cock ring around the base of your lover's cock and either turn the attached torpedo downward to stimulate his perineum or upward to stimulate your clitoris (and he'll also feel the vibrations on the base of his penis).

Leading Him by the Balls

Taking the traditional cock ring to another level, a cock leash consists of a ring that goes around your lover's whole package and has a leash attached. Not only does controlling his cock give you a feeling of empowerment, the gentle tugging sensations also feel really good to your man.

A Stretch of Imagination

Ball stretchers are little cuffs made of leather or cloth that are attached directly above the testicles and around the scrotum and closed with snaps. While the name of this toy may cause men to wince, once they experience this plaything, they realize the hands-free pulling sensation is to die for!

> Let your lover know his kinky confidence turns you on, and suggest that he wear one of these items under his clothes so you can *discover* them during foreplay.

SOME TOYS ARE CREATED EQUAL

While some sex playthings are gender specific, and though any toy can be creatively incorporated into sex play, some toys were created for simultaneous enjoyment. Here are some of our divas' favorite equal-opportunity toys.

Nipple Clamps

We're not talking about the wooden clothespins of yore, we mean the newly fashioned fun and stylish clamps that give nipple nerve-endings endless pleasure. For nipple-sensitive men and women, these items are a must-have! Choose the perfect ones for you.

Tweezer Clamps

These are the best nipple clamps for novices. They are the most comfortable, and the tension can be adjusted simply by sliding the small ring closer or farther away from the nipple. Also, the narrow, curved, plastic-covered-wire ends close around the base of the nipple, so they leave the tip standing up at attention. This allows easy access for licking and teasing as your or your lover's nipples are squeezed in satisfaction!

Clove Clamps

For the more advanced sex-toy player, these nipple clamps are big, sturdy, and slightly intimidating. The pressure is not adjustable and is generally hard and rough. The gripper pads consist of mini-rubber disks with stimulating bumps, which also help keep the clamps firmly in place without abrading the skin. Also, there is a chain attached to this nipple toy. The dominant partner can tug on the chain to increase tension and enhance nipple pleasure. Oh behave!

Kitty Clamps

Again, this is not a beginner's toy. These alligator-type clamps have adjusting screws, limiting how tightly they can be fastened. But here's the kinky kicker—cylindrical weights are attached. Turn the dial and the clamps hum, gently stimulating the captive nipples. Up the dial, and the clamps purr with more passion and make nipples dance with delight!

Clamp It, Baby!

Now that you've decided what toy tickles your fancy, it's time to learn the basics of how to use them to their full advantage.

- Make sure nipples are erect before clamping on these sex toys. Stroke, caress, suck, kiss, lick, and squeeze them to get them to pinched perfection!
- Start by clamping as much flesh as possible and, over time, begin clamping less and less. As with any new adventure,

you should advance gradually, allowing your lover to get comfortable with the new sensations the toy imparts.

- As you become more proficient with nipple clamps, you can clamp less flesh, to create more pressure and intensify the sensations. DO NOT clip only the tip of the nipple, however. The sensation will be too strong for pleasure, and you can risk tearing the skin.
- Watch the time, and ensure you don't clamp nipples for more than ten to fifteen minutes at a time. Clamps restrict blood flow to the nipples and surrounding tissues. Sexual arousal can mask pain, so your lover may not realize that damage is being done. Also, the longer nipple clamps are on, the more they hurt coming off, since blood will rush back to the area. Find a happy medium length of time.
- Once nipples are clamped, tease them with feathers, silk scarves, and your tongue for additional sensation.

> Re-emphasize to your lover that sex toys are for additional pleasure. Don't let him sit on the sidelines as the toy does its work. Let him know you still need him in the game to achieve a touchdown. Sports-oriented dirty talk will get him standing at attention!

Anal Sex Toys

Anal sex toys are butts above the rest, because the sensations they produce are unique and often more powerful than you can get with other toys. This is because your anus has more nerve endings than your clit, nipples, and the tip of his penis all added together. So any anal play provides immense sexual satisfaction. Plus, the experience is something you both can enjoy since you both have amazing anuses to indulge in. So dive into this pleasure zone and cum through the back door with these porn-star favorites:

Butt Plugs

Butt plugs are designed to fit snugly and comfortably into your anus. They are typically cone-shaped, with a flared base that prevents them from slipping into your rectum. You can use them for butt play, to stimulate the endless nerve endings in your anus, or during vaginal sex, to give you the sensation of being completely filled by your lover, thus making the urge to orgasm that much stronger. An additional plus for him: the bulge in the middle of a butt plug stimulates his prostate.

Anal Beads

Anal beads come in all different colors, sizes, and styles. Like pearls, they are knotted together into place along a string and have a ring at one end. You insert the beads into your or your lover's anus and one by one, pull the beads out. The sensations of the beads going in and coming out of your anus causes your sphincter muscles to contract, which feels incredible and can greatly intensify orgasms in both men and women.

Learn more about the history of sex toys at the Museum of Sex in New York City. Not only will you get an educational tour of your favorite pastime, the visuals will get you hungry and horny to make some sexual history of your own!

See It to Believe It!

Don't have time to visit a museum but want to have an educational introduction to sex toys? Here are some favorite videos to get revved up for some sex-toy play.

Nina Hartley's Guide to Sex Toys—Adam and Eve Productions, 2000, 87 minutes

Bend Over Boyfriend—Fatale Video, 1998, 60 minutes

Bonus Tip: Always remember: Zero fear equals fantastic fornication. If you are wary of any sex toy, start playing with it gradually until you are comfortable enough to enjoy it fully. Those who are slow and steady win the randy race!

Director's Cut

 ## HOW TO SORT OUT THE GOOD, THE BAD, AND THE VERY, VERY SEXY

> Sex is a conversation carried out by other means.
>
> —Peter Ustinov

Video directors have to focus on what looks smoking hot, what steams up the camera lens, and what tightens the crew's pants. This involves editing film reels so that each shot is just as naughty as the next.

While it may seem that you and your lover don't have the luxury of editing out the sex moves you tried that were more tepid than sizzling, you actually do. Couples who discuss their sex lives outside the bedroom have the opportunity to cut what doesn't work for them sexually and keep what does.

Here are a few ideas for critiquing your randy romps.

TALK TO ME, BABY

Giving confidence-boosting constructive criticism is not as hard as it sounds. Follow these carnal communication commandments:

- Never say anything negative right after sex. Both lovers can feel very vulnerable and sensitive after coitus.

- Always whisper reassuring tidbits into each other's ears to commend one another like "That was wonderful," "You are amazing," or even a simple, breathless "Thank You." Always wait until at least the morning after to let your lover know that a certain move didn't really work for you.
- Always emphasize the positive, and your lover will be sure to get the hint. For example, say "It drives me crazy when you lick my pussy that way." This will let him know you crave more tongue action when he's going down on you. Or "When you pulled my hair last night, it really fired me up. Could you do more of that?"
- Never make light of something you are unsatisfied with. If you make a joke, such as, "You know that thing you tried last night? That was...*interesting*," then it seems you are making fun of your lover's lovemaking capabilities. Instead, be genuine and gentle. Sincerity generates better steamy results.

Silence Is Golden

Though honesty is the best policy generally, sometimes a little white lie can keep a new relationship red-hot. Approach new relationships like a blank canvas, and don't taint them with any mishaps from your past. Here are some items you should *never* discuss with your lover:

How many people have you slept with?

There is no right answer to this question. If his number is higher than yours, you may be upset or freak out. If his is lower than yours, you may feel judged. Do not risk an uncomfortable conversation based on the rare chance that your numbers may be the same. If you must inquire about your lover's past sexual experiences, ask him what his first sexual experience was like, or what fantasy he has that he's never had fulfilled. This will give you insight into his sexual past without having to bring any numbers into play. This also gives you the ability to become the lover who will perform his unfulfilled fantasy.

Have you ever faked an orgasm?

No matter how honest you may be feeling when your partner pops this question, never say yes! Even if you vow you'll never do it again, every time you're riding the waves to bliss, he'll doubt your sincerity. Don't even admit you've faked it with previous lovers. The idea that you have faked it before makes him think you could fake it again. Just make a private promise to yourself to never fool your lover again.

That great thing your ex did.

Your lover doesn't want to envision you kissing someone else, never mind fucking someone else. And they *never* want to hear how a previous lover drove you crazy in bed in ways that he cannot. Your partner wants to be your best lover ever, not a runner-up in a previous conquest's shadow. So if you desire a technique your current lover has yet to perform, simply ask for it. There is no need to explain the origin of this carnal request.

Have you ever cheated?

Even if you have never cheated on your current lover, the admission that you have cheated in the past can cause your partner to mistrust you. This knowledge can make him doubt your every move, become suspicious and controlling, and ultimately ruin the entire relationship. Begin a new leaf and leave your cheating ways behind you, but never admit any past transgressions.

As they say, great sex is built on trust, but phenomenal sex is built on trust and a few necessary omissions.

LIGHTS, CAMERA, ACTION!

Since you are the ultimate sex star, why not use a camera to heat up your sex life—and to help critique it with your lover? What better way to finesse your lovemaking skills than watching yourself in the act? It's both fun and educational.

Take these tips for taking a camera into your hands, and make some spectacular porn of your own. Always be sure to establish trust with your partner before you begin shooting.

• Before you start, talk about the direction in which you want to take your movie. Do you want to re-create a kinky classic, or invent something more fun and frisky? How about something more red-hot and steamy?

• Be sure to have some props on hand—silk sheets, fruit and chocolate, your favorite sex toys—to incorporate into your film, based on a theme you choose.

• Remember that this may not be the first time either of you has played porn star. Do not be disappointed if your lover seems to know what he is doing. Use his experience to heighten your own pleasure.

- Run a screen test before you start filming. Take tasteful digital pictures of each other. This way you both can become more comfortable in front of a lens and see how fantastic you look onscreen. You can build trust between you when you hit the "delete" button together.

- Though we've said you should never fake an orgasm, you both can do a little extra moaning and groaning for the sake of the camera. A dramatic soundtrack can make the whole experience that more intoxicating.

- Never use the close-up option on the camera. Raw footage will pick up all the flaws that are airbrushed out of commercial pornography. Use a wider angle to capture your tryst. Also, if possible, hook the camera up to your television so you can view the footage while you are in the midst of filming. A quick look to the left and you can ensure the sex is H-O-T. Plus, it offers the same tantalizing visuals as if you were checking your romp out in the mirror.

- Make sure you get the money shot. Talk beforehand about where he will cum, to avoid any uncomfortable mishaps.

- View the video a few times, but always remember to play it safe and destroy the footage together. There is too much to risk of the film landing in the wrong hands, and besides, it gives you a chance to make another frisky film sometime soon!

PLAYING PORN STAR

If you lack the porn-star gene but still have a deep-rooted desire to perform for your lover, we have a few obscene options for you to explore. You can have fun playing pretend-porn, making up sexy monikers for each other and creating arousing alter egos.

The act of talking about sex in a playful manner can help you and your lover eventually become more comfortable talking about more serious lovemaking matters. It opens the lines of communication, which is the key to better sex!

Say My Name

Create kinky names for your lover and yourself. Follow these tips on inventing the best name for you—but remember, this may be something that gets screamed night after night!

- For those who lack carnal creativity, one simple way to create your porn-star name is to combine the name of your first pet and your first street address. "Shadow Robinwood"—Oh my!
- Riff on an element of your personality to give your porn-star name some deeper meaning. "Mystery," "Sunshine," and "Felicity" are just a few saucy suggestions.
- Put some wordplay into your porn play. Pick a sensuous name that begins with the same letter as your own first name. Think "Voluptuous Valerie," "Juicy Jennifer," or "Luscious Laura."
- Incorporate some of your own personal tastes into your porn name. If your style is more conservative and classy, go with something like "Clarissa." If you have a more modern taste, think "Mona."
- You can even steal the name of your favorite musician, artist, author, or poet. What you may lack in creativity, you can always make up for in kinkiness.

Your Sexy Signature Move

A sultry signature move can define who you are sexually. To really channel your inner sex goddess, you need to identify a move that will make you legendary.

Discuss with your lover what you'd be famous for if you were a porn star. You may be surprised that a simple move that you perform rocks his world! Or you may learn that that thing you do with your tongue doesn't turn him on so much. It's a great way to critique both of your sexual techniques in a light-hearted manner.

After your discussion, have your lover assign one signature move to you, and you assign one to your lover in return. Then you can both prove how well you perform it during your next raunchy romp! You may even win the erotic equivalent to an Oscar—your lover's standing ovation.

Playing Director and Actor

As we've established, an open camera lens does not always inspire open legs. But once you've established a porn-star name and a sexy signature move, you're ready to take turns with your lover controlling a make-believe movie set and stealing the luscious limelight.

Director: Do a fake photo shoot, and make your lover strike erotic poses while you click away. Or, while you're getting down and dirty, call out directions to your lover to compose the hottest "shots." You can also choose the setting, the clothing, the music, and the toys!

Star: Get ready for your close-up. Develop a classy character who's in touch with her carnal side, and only enact scenarios that you feel would be true to that personality. Follow the director's ribald requests, or perform acts all on your own. A star is born!

If you're too shy to perform in front of the camera but want to watch the action as it unfolds, place a mirror strategically next to you as you have sex. Watching yourself in the reflection will allow you to critique your lovemaking skills later on and will make the sex even hotter right now.

See It to Believe It!

Here are some educational videos that concentrate on how openly discussing your fantasies with your long-term lover is key for exceptional sex:

Sexual Ecstasy for Couples—Libido Films, 1997, 62 minutes

Ordinary Couples, Extraordinary Sex series—Sinclair Intimacy Institute, 1994, 60 minutes each. Series includes:

- ***Discovering Extraordinary Sex***
- ***Getting Creative with Sex***
- ***Keeping Sex Extraordinary***

Bonus Tip: Always remember: Carnal communication with your lover is just as important as the consummation itself.

The Ultimate Visual Stimulation

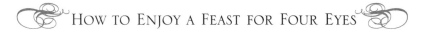

HOW TO ENJOY A FEAST FOR FOUR EYES

> The porn industry is a lot of fun, and people shouldn't be afraid. The industry is only going to get bigger and more mainstream.
>
> —Johnna Long

Despite puritanical popular belief, pornography is not filthy, and watching it does not make you "one of those girls." It can be used as an essential guide to sex. It can be used to learn a few new tantalizing tricks. Or it can be used solely as a visual stimulus to heighten your sexual experience. According to a *Ladies Home Journal* survey, 47 percent of women report using pornography to intensify and improve sex with their lovers. Research done by a law professor at Northwestern University also suggests that an increased access to porn on the Internet may be one of the reasons that the incidence of reported rape has declined 85 percent since the 1970s.

But in the end, the proof of the percentages is in the viewing. Pick up some porn next time you're feeling horny, and you'll discover that while some movies still portray women as objects, most (especially those directed by women) transcend stereotypes and offer storylines with sex interlaced into them. You'll see a new world of classy porn.

Watching porn with your lover can open the gates to sexual communication. You can talk about what you're viewing, and learn about each other's preferences and boundaries as they come up in the films. You might even discover a fantastic fantasy that your lover has that you never knew about. And now knowing that you have the porn stars' secrets up your sleeves, you'll be able to fulfill that fantasy with confidence.

Our final porn-star suggestions focus on how to use porn to spice up a lackluster relationship (or heighten a red-hot one) and act out some sizzling sex scenes of your own.

LET'S GIVE THEM SOMETHING TO TALK ABOUT

The first step toward watching porn together is first discussing the idea together. Bring up your desire to indulge in some visual eye-candy in a comfortable environment, such as

- While cuddling on the couch
- During an intimate dinner
- Taking a walk together
- When confessing a sexual fantasy.

Or, if you find it difficult to bring up directly, you could watch a mainstream movie that has some hot sex scenes, and comment on the steamy interchanges that interest you. Here is a list of favorites.

- *Basic Instinct* (Director's Cut)
- *Better Than Chocolate*
- *Body of Evidence*

- *Boogie Nights*
- *Bound*
- *Crash* (Director's Cut)
- *The Fluffer*
- *Henry and June*
- *Holy Smoke*
- *The Hunger*
- *Jade*
- *Kama Sutra*
- *Last Tango in Paris*
- *$9\frac{1}{2}$ Weeks*
- *Secretary*

After viewing, casually bring up how you'd like to watch more scenes or films like that with your partner. More than likely, he will be thrilled at the idea of using porn to heighten your sex life.

SEX SHOPPING LIST

Now that you've discussed viewing porn, it's time to choose some together. Since most people have different tastes, it is essential to discuss what kinds of porn you would like to add to your sex life. Pay attention to what types of videos you and your lover are drawn to. Notice if the videos you or he pick up have a similar theme, such as girl-on-girl action, or foot fetishes. You may learn a thing or two about yourselves in the selection process.

Here are some ideas for finding the types of films that are right for both of you.

- Check out online porn websites, since they often have

summaries and viewer reviews. These allow you to investigate which genres, themes, and categories work for you both in the privacy of your own home.

- Visit a local porn store together and browse the aisles. You might find some naughty goodies to accompany your video as well.
- You can also go to your local video store and slip behind the black curtain to check out some white-hot films for yourselves (many porn stores have video booths in which you can watch films).
- Check out the lists at the end of this chapter. They categorize porn by genre and kinky specialty and give director synopses and tidbits of information for each film.

INTERACTIVE PORN

While simply talking about porn can steam up your relationship, watching porn together can ignite some serious fireworks. Here are some porn-star suggestions for things to try next time you're cuddled on the couch with your lover watching something steamy:

- While you are wrapped up together in a blanket or throw, watch a film with your hands in each other's laps. Let your hands wander to yourself or your lover as you react to what is happening on the screen. Covering up what your hands are doing will highlight the naughty nature of your activities.
- Mimic the positions of the actors onscreen as they are copulating. The best positions to try are Reverse Cowgirl, Spooning, or Doggy Style. This way you can still both view your frisky film as you are getting it on!

- Take turns: Give oral sex to your lover as he is watching the DVD, and vice versa.

SEX PLAY

When you press "play" on the DVD player, how about playing some sexy games during the viewing that'll guarantee a steamy night?

- Try to watch the entire movie without touching yourself or your lover. After the credits roll, assume the characters of two of the stars and let the games begin!
- Kiss your lover every time a porn star moans onscreen, or grab his cock every time she takes off an item of clothing. If you don't like these rules, make up your own—the possibilities are endless!
- Turn on a video right around the time that your lover normally gets home from work. Pretend to be caught in the act!
- Tie your lover to a chair and tell him he *must* watch the movie. While he watches, do some of the naughty things happening on screen to him. Let your bad-girl persona rule!
- Play a porn DVD but turn the sound off. Intensify the visual stimulation by seducing your lover with a striptease or oral sex.

XXX RATED

With naughty new thoughts running through your head and your lover sitting right next to you, all you need now is the proper visual stimulation to get going! The problem is, with so many movies to choose from, finding one that is just right can be daunting, and you may end up purchasing or renting films you strongly dislike. To help you find ones that will rock your world, here's a list of our porn-stars' favorites, by genre.

For Porn Virgins

For couples who have never viewed porn together, here are a few great films to help you ease into the idea. They are not too graphic, violent, or extreme, but they have sex-driven plots and voluptuous visuals to make the sparks fly between you.

History of the Blue Movie—Dir. Alex DeRenzy, 1983, 108 minutes

This film is more of a documentary than a feature film. It is a collection of early erotic films that are entertaining and exciting.

Barbara Broadcast—Dir. Henry Paris, 1977, 90 minutes

Annette Haven plays a celebrity call-girl and best-selling sex author who has a secret admirer. Kinky and romantic, this film is way above average.

Amanda by Night—Dir. Robert McCallum, 1982, 95 minutes

This film features Veronica Hart, one of our highlighted female directors, before she had taken up directing. Hart plays a high-class prostitute trying to turn over a new leaf when she suddenly finds herself in the middle of a murder.

Amanda by Night 2—Dir. Jack Remy, 1988, 85 minutes

A sequel actually worthy of its predecessor, this film incorporates mystery, murder, and sex all in one steamy package.

Thighs Wide Open—Dir. Fred J. Lincoln, 2001, 95 minutes
Chloe is married to a man who openly cheats on her, and she shuts herself off sexually—until she meets the right group of people! Watch for the hot staircase encounter!

Sunset Stripped—Dir. Veronica Hart, 2002, 137 minutes
This film pays homage to *Sunset Boulevard* and is full of real female orgasms and mesmerizing sex. Plus, the women call the shots in all these sex scenes. What could be better than that?!

One Size Fits All—Dir. Candida Royalle, 1998, 79 minutes
Think *The Sisterhood of the Traveling Pants*, but here there is a hot dress and genuine sensual sex. The film stars two of our favorite divas, Nina Hartley and Candida Royalle.

My Surrender—Dir. Candida Royalle, 1996, 82 minutes
This sexy drama centers on a woman who films couples having sex but remains alone because of her own intimacy issues. Then a mysterious man enters her life and changes everything.

Love's Passion—Dir. Veronica Hart, 1998, 120 minutes
This film intertwines the present day with the Civil War period. It is romantic, tender, and raw—just the way sex should be!

Looking In—Dir. Paul Thomas, 2002, 108 minutes
A compelling film, this piece looks more like a mainstream movie than porn. Thomas interlaces explicit sex scenes with a rich plot involving voyeurism and infidelity. Keep an eye out for the hot-wax scene—breathtaking!

The Hottest Bid—Dir. Deborah Shames, 1995, 90 minutes
This film may be the perfect way to introduce porn to a shy lover. A middle-aged couple attends a charity auction where women bid for dates with a sexy guy. Nice, light, soft-core romance.

The Gift—Dir. Candida Royalle, 1997, 87 minutes
The theme of this film: sensual lovemaking!

Ecstatic Moments—Dir. Marianna Beck and Jack Hafferkamp, 1999, 78 minutes
Three separate women indulge in their wildest sexual fantasies. This film includes S/M, sex toys, and other kinky endeavors.

Female Director Highlight—Candida Royalle

Candida Royalle is a porn-star-turned-director who keeps women specifically in mind when she makes her films. Royalle started Femme Productions in 1984, and unlike many production companies whose films focus on male orgasms and masculine pleasure, she began directing porn films that address female fantasies and indulge feminine visual needs. Her erotic films portray women as sexual role-models and focus on plot and character. That's not to say she doesn't get raunchy, but she also reveals a sensual side of pornography. Many of her beginning works were more soft-core, but her later endeavors have become more explicit. Most plots are cute and romantic, but the sex is laced with carnal chemistry, and she never undermines the focus on fulfilling female viewers' sexual needs. Her films are very realistic, avoid genital close-ups, and show men ejaculating inside women (rather than featuring "money shots").

The Elements of Great Sex

For the more porn-savvy couple, here are some great flicks to watch to get your kicks:

Believe It Or Not—Dir. Paul Thomas, 2001, 106 minutes and ***Believe It Or Not 2***—Dir. Paul Thomas, 2001, 70 minutes

These films can open the lines of communication with your lover in a fun and flirty way. In them, Thomas hooks porn stars up to a lie detector and asks them to tell him their wildest sexual encounter, then has them re-enact it for the camera. Some stars are telling the truth, some are not. It's up to you to determine which is which!

Fantasy Island

Films that explore fantasies are one of the best genres for couples to watch together. They explore fantasy and role-playing and inspire viewers to bring some movie magic into their own lovemaking. The artistic costumes, imaginative scripts, and beautiful settings will also get viewers' creative juices flowing!

Taken—Dir. Veronica Hart, 2001, 142 minutes

Ginger Lynn plays a woman who is abducted and then seduced by a tall, dark, and handsome stranger. Full of realistic characters and passionate lovemaking, this film is at the top of the female fantasy genre.

Dream Quest—Dir. Brad Armstrong, 1999, 100 minutes

This film is the ultimate fantasy porn. With its *Lord of the Rings* style, it has equally impressive effects, mind-blowing sex, and a great spanking scene.

The Masseuse—Dir. Paul Thomas, 1990, 85 minutes

The Masseuse 2—Dir. Paul Thomas, 1994, 120 minutes

The Masseuse 3—Dir. Paul Thomas, 1998, 120 minutes

Everyone's favorite fantasy! Watch as men are seduced by masseuses who take the ultimate pride in their work! Well-drafted scripts, full of great acting.

The Marquis De Sade—Dir. Joe D'Amato, 1995, 85 minutes

This film follows the tale of the master pervert and contains wonderful period costumes, intense sex scenes, and great chemistry among the actors.

Flashpoint—Dir. Brad Armstrong, 1997, 120 minutes

Want to indulge your fireman fantasies? What about your firewoman fantasies? This film follows Jenna Jameson as a hot-to-trot firefighter searching for love and scorching sex.

Autobiography of a Flea—Dir. Sharon MacNight, 1984, 93 minutes

One of the most talked about fantasy-porn films in the industry, this flick features a young girl so beautiful that all men who see her want to rape her. However, once they think they've conquered her, she quickly turns on them and fucks them with fiery lust.

Female Director Highlight—Tina Tyler

Another famous porn-diva-turned-director, Tina Tyler directs quality films with quantity sex! She uses wonderful plots to maneuver through fantastic sexual acts. Just check out *Tina Tyler's Going Down* for proof! And her girl-on-girl and fellatio scenes are rated the best in tinsel-town.

Mainstream Movie Mimic

For those of you who want something familiar in your porn, these next films are for you. Their plots are based on great mainstream movies and television series, but the sex is one hundred percent mouth-wateringly original.

Shakespeare

Hamlet—Dir. Joe D'Amato, 1996, 76 minutes
This randy remake was filmed on location and includes incredible costumes and a very attractive cast.

Desperate Housewives

Bliss—Dir. Antonio Passolini, 1999, 120 minutes
Juli Ashton is the perfect wife, at least until her sexual compulsiveness ruins her marriage. The acting is outstanding in this film, and the camerawork is cutting-edge.

The Other Side of Julie—Dir. Anthony Riverton, 1981, 83 minutes
John Leslie's wife decides to find her own sexual satisfaction after she discovers her husband is having one affair after another. The film is sensuous and the sex is unhurried.

Bad Wives—Dir. Paul Thomas, 1997, 147 minutes
Two wives are tired of the restrictions of marriage and discover the delights of infidelity and kinky sex. This film is jam-packed with anal sex scenes.

Bad Wives 2—Dir. Paul Thomas, 2001, 106 minutes
Different wives. And a lot more trouble. These wives are

in prison for attempting to murder their horrible husbands. Watch as they try to seduce their way out from behind bars.

I Dream of Jeannie

I Dream of Jenna—Dir. Justin Sterling, 2002, 120 minutes

Jenna Jameson plays a genie that grants everyone's wishes! Watch for the award-winning girl-on-girl action scene.

My Fair Lady

Opening of Misty Beethoven—Dir. Henry Paris, 1976, 86 minutes

Researching a book he's writing, Jamie Gillis seeks out a prostitute and attempts to make her into a refined, respectable call girl. It has all the elements of good porn: great acting, wonderful directing, and stars who really enjoy getting it on!

Dracula

Dracula Exotic—Dir. Warren Evans, 1980, 98 minutes

The count is fleeing to America to evade Hungarian tax collectors and finds hot sex, fantastic fetishes, and eager victims along the way.

Jekyll and Hyde

Jekyll and Hyde—Dir. Paul Thomas, 2000, 93 minutes

This film is full of Victorian dresses, sexy corsets, and mysterious drama. The majority of the cast is European, which means there are all kinds of astonishing natural bodies, wonderful acting, and great fucking!

Thelma and Louise

Anything That Moves—Dir. John Leslie, 1992, 76 minutes
Two strippers go on a sexual rampage. Great sex and exotic pole dancing ensue. What more is there to love?!

Clockwork Orange

Clockwork Orgy—Dir. Nic Cramer, 1996, 75 minutes
This film showcases a gang of cruel, horny women roaming the streets and having sex with whomever they please—many times without consent. It emphasizes female dominance and power. Oh how sweet it is!

Fight Club

Club Sin—Dir. Antonio Passolini, 2001, 99 minutes
Two women start an underground sex club where women use men as a way to emphasize their dominance.

Cinderella

Sinful Rella—Dir. Veronica Hart, 2002, 88 minutes
This film approaches the Cinderella theme with modern porn humor. Lighthearted and flirty, the sex scenes concentrate on female satisfaction just as much as male.

Female Director Highlight—Marianna Beck

Marianna Beck partners with Jeff Hafferkamp to direct some of the most realistic porn films in the industry. Her plots are simple and her actors are completely natural. Plus, her stars always have intense onscreen chemistry and the greatest unconventional sex. If you're itching to learn some seriously racy sack skills, check out this directing duo.

Cult Classics

Want to be a porn connoisseur? Watch these cult classics to see where it all began. These groundbreaking films not only brought porn into the mainstream, they also helped open the lines of sexual communication. You'll be sure to learn an erotic thing or two!

The Devil in Miss Jones—Dir. Gerald Damiano, 1972, 62 minutes

Justice Jones, an old spinster, commits suicide in her bathroom to only discover she has gone to purgatory and can barter with the devil for more time—as long as she lives her life consumed by lust. Every sex scene is enjoyable and refreshing.

Debbie Does Dallas—Dir. Jim Clark, 1978, 83 minutes

Debbie is a head cheerleader who, in order to pay her own way to go to Dallas to be on a professional cheerleading team, gives head and other oral services for a fee. This film is fun, kitschy, and campy!

Alice in Wonderland—Dir. Bud Townsend, 1976, 81 minutes

This is a porn musical masterpiece! The film features great acting, beautiful costumes, and wonderful cinematography as the characters bump and grind their way through Carroll's classic story. Avoid the soft-core R-rated version and look for the X-rated one.

Caligula—Dir. Tinto Brass, 1979, 148 minutes
This film features major movie stars including Peter O'Toole and Helen Mirren. The story follows the life of Emperor Caligula of Rome, whose spiral into madness because of the horrors he inflicted on others was legendary. Watch for the improved lesbian scene.

Behind the Green Door—Dir. Artie and Jim Mitchell, 1973, 68 minutes
This film is not for the faint of heart since it contains some themes that continue to shock today's audiences, such as abduction and forced sexual penetration. These controversial sex scenes can spark carnal communication with your partner, however.

Deep Throat—Dir. Jim Clark, 1978, 83 minutes
This cult classic revolves around Linda Lovelace, who discovers that her clitoris is located in her throat. Deep-throated blowjobs ensue.

Cinderella—Dir. Michael Pataki, 1977, 78 minutes
Another musical with a lot of punch! This film has sizzling sex, great musical numbers, and humorous porno caricatures of Cinderella characters. A true sexual satire if you ever saw one!

Café Flesh—Dir. Rinse Dream, 1983, 90 minutes
It's 1984, porn-style. This film is set in the future, in the aftermath of World War III and the "nuclear kiss" that has made ninety-nine percent of humanity into "sex negatives." The remaining one percent must perform sexual acts as entertainment to the public. The story follows a negative couple through their intimate journey of self-discovery.

Female Intuition

Just as females crave different sexual acts than males, they also crave different porn, so we asked our porn divas to list their favorite movies. Next time the night is all about you, pop in one of these DVDs and play sweet 'n' sexy.

Appossionata—Dir. Asia Carrera and Bude Lee, 1998, 92 minutes

In one of the most acclaimed porn films in the industry, Asia Carrera plays a young pianist passionate about music and love. Veronica Hart, one of our favorite female directors, also stars.

Cabin Fever—Dir. Deborah Shames, 1995, 45 minutes

In order to get away from busy city life, a woman retreats into her cabin to concentrate on her art work. There she meets a handsome handyman. The rest is romantic history. This film is soft-core with a sexy edge.

Revelations—Dir. Candida Royalle, 1992, 120 minutes

This movie is set in a future where pleasurable sex is prohibited. The plot follows one girl who dares discover the truth. This film focuses on female pleasure and almost seems more like a sophisticated R-rated movie than porn.

Looking In—Dir. Paul Thomas, 2002, 108 minutes

Viewing this film is like watching a great Hollywood movie, with lots of hot sex laced into the plot. A young couple moves into their new home to find that their neighbors harbor a dark and kinky side. Explore voyeurism, infidelity, and some forbidden fetishes from the comfort of your own couch. And keep an eye out for the steamy hot-wax scene.

Lisa—Dir. Kris Kramski, 2000, 1997 minutes

Lisa is a beautiful girl who has engaged in a tryst with her selfish, abusive boyfriend and his friend. Once she decides to leave him behind for treating her so badly, she embarks on a journey of self-discovery and pulsating, passionate sex.

Emmanuelle—Dir. Just Jaeckin, 1973, 94 minutes

Emmanuelle is married to an ambassador. When she expresses her weariness with their relationship, he tells her to explore the benefits of an open relationship. And she does! While the film is very well made, Emmanuelle is often cast in submissive roles and used for men's pleasure. This cult classic is best remembered for the scene in which a woman smokes a cigarette with her vagina.

Honorable Mentions

Three Daughters—Dir. Candida Royalle, 1987, 80 minutes

This film is directed by Candida Royalle, so you know it's going to be good!

The New Devil in Miss Jones—Dir. Paul Thomas, 2005, 108 minutes

This porn flick features Jenna Jameson in a modern remake of the cult classic!

Female Director Highlight—Veronica Hart

Veronica Hart is one of the first female porn-vixen-turned-directors to focus on the female characters in her films and on their erotic experiences and pleasures. She fearlessly explores all female fantasies, from romance to rough sex and even down-and-dirty gangbanging. She even approaches complex and controversial female fantasy plots, such as female-rape fantasies, and showcases them in a simple and romantic manner. Her plots are rich and her scripts are tight. Add top-shelf porn stars to the mix and you've got yourself one great porno film!

Sex, Sex, Sex

Want to view hardcore sex without the bells and whistles of tinsel-town? These films are your hot tickets.

V: The Hot One—Dir. Robert McCallum, 1984, 89 minutes
Annette Haven is married to a high-powered lawyer, and while she may appear cool and sophisticated, she is looking for some hot and heavy sexcapades.

3 A.M.—Dir. Robert McCallum, 1975, 90 minutes
Georgina Spelvin plays a woman having an affair with her brother-in-law. Conflicts within the family arise, while great sex dominates this cult-classic film.

An American Girl in Paris—Dir. Kris Kramski, 1998, 69 minutes
While this film has little-to-no plot, the insatiable amount of steamy sex makes up for it. The audience follows an American girl who travels to Paris alone and loses her wallet and passport and must survive. It is a sensational sex film, shot entirely on location.

Sex—Dir. Michael Ninn, 1993 and *Sex 2: Fate*—Dir. Michael Ninn, 1994, 85 minutes
Celebrity life is not all glitz and glamour. This film centers on sex celebrities as they delve deeper into the deceit and darkness of the film industry. Stylish sex scenes are paired with excellent acting.

Michael Ninn's Perfect—Dir. Michael Ninn, 2002, 129 minutes
This film is what porn movie magic is all about! With its *Matrix*-like special effects and great sexual core, it's perfect all around. With anal sex, and some boot-licking fun, it's got a little something for everyone.

The Zone—Dir. Paul Thomas, 1998, 90 minutes
See the world of a sex club through the eyes of a recent divorcée. With its searing sex scenes and sexually dominant women, this film is sophisticated and stylish.

Fetish Favorites

For couples who want to introduce fetishes and S/M into their sex life but need something to push them over the erotic edge, here are some great films to watch together. Just keep in mind that most S/M movies do not include sex. They do, however, push the pulsating envelope.

Lesbian/Girl-On-Girl S/M

The Black Glove—Dir. Maria Beatty, 1996, 30 minutes
A young submissive woman will do anything to please her lover, including indulging in spanking, foot worshiping, and hot-wax play.

Dark Paradise—Dir. Ernest Greene, 1999, 89 minutes
This film revolves around Japanese rope bondage and some classic pony-girl services.

The Elegant Spanking—Dir. Maria Beatty, 1995, 30 minutes
This elegant spanking film is also elegantly made. The

classic black-and-white feature tells the story of the punishment of a housemaid by her mistress. It includes dominant/submissive role-playing, urination, and a wonderfully elegant spanking.

S/M For Everyone!

Art of Bondage Series—Dir. M. Zabel, 1998, approximately 60 minutes

These films cover a wide range of S/M styles, from spankings to nipple clamps. Plus, the actors are clad in the latest S/M fashions and fetish gear. A feast for your eyes!

Portrait of a Dominatrix—Dir. Ernest Greene, 1998, 60 minutes

Mistress Midori, the ultimate dominatrix of our time, reveals her sexual appetite through various stages of her life. She begins by demonstrating how she seduced her college professor and ends by showing how she now turns men into puppies with cock and ball torture. Naughty boys, listen up!

Seduction: The Cruel Woman—Dir. Monika Treut, Elfi Mickesch, 1989, 84 minutes

This film does not fully indulge in S/M or fetish games but deserves an honorable mention as it beautifully portrays submissive and dominant role-playing between very well developed characters. Filmed in black-and-white with subtle tonal variations, this film is perfect for the art crazed.

Testify My Love—Dir. Maria Beatty, 1999, 42 minutes

A young man wants to marry the woman of his dreams, but

she first makes him pass a ritual set of tests, including sexual humiliation, blindfolding and bondage, and losing his "virginity."

Thank You, Mistress—Dir. Marianna Beck and Jack Hafferkamp, 2000, 35 minutes

A woman fulfills her lover's S/M fantasy and gives him to a cruel and sexy dominatrix. The sex play among all three of them brings the couple closer then they've ever been. A must-see to view with your lover if you want to bring a slice of S/M into your love life.

S/M with Sex—A Double Feature

The Fashionistas—Dir. John "Buttman" Stagliano, 2002, 280 minutes

Clamps, clips, whips, chains...Oh my! This film actually indulges in both S/M activities *and* sex.

The Story of O—Dir. Just Jaekin, 1984, 96 minutes

A young woman, called simply "O," must do anything her master asks to prove her loyalty and submission. Full of all the classic S/M accoutrements and hot steamy sex scenes.

Female Director Highlight—Nina Hartley

Not only is Nina Hartley a performer-turned-director, she's also a former professional nurse. So when she gives you tips, tricks, and titillating tidbits about how to make your sex life better, she knows what she's talking about! Given her background, she also tends to feature strong feminist viewpoints in her films. We've highlighted her educational videos throughout this book, but her feature films are just as saucy. If you and your honey are in sexploration mode, pick up one of her flicks!

Genre Orgy

#1 films in each of the following steamy genres:

Toys
Justice: Nothing to Hide 2—Dir. Paul Thomas, 1994, 90 minutes

Masturbation
Tina Tyler's Going Down—Dir. Tina Tyler, 2002, 74 minutes

Threesomes/Orgies
Façade—Dir. Paul Thomas, 2000, 100 minutes

Blowjobs
Unreal—Dir. Antonio Passolini, 2001, 112 minutes

International
Flamenco Ecstasy—Dir. Joe D'Amato, 1997, 70 minutes (Spanish)

Humorous
Mobster's Wife—Dir. Paul Thomas, 1998, 120 minutes

Bonus Tip: Always remember: Porn cannot taint your sex life, it can only enrich it with new experiences, so always keep your mind open as you watch these visual treats together.